Solutions Manual to Accompany

Sampling of Populations

Solutions Manual to Accompany

Sampling of Populations

Methods and Applications

Fourth Edition

Paul S. Levy
RTI International
Statistical Research Division
Research Triangle Park, NC

Stanley Lemeshow
The Ohio State University
College of Public Health
Columbus, OH

Prepared by

Erinn M. Hade
The Ohio State University
Center for Biostatistics
Columbus, OH

Amy K. Ferketich
The Ohio State University
College of Public Health
Columbus, OH

WILEY

A JOHN WILEY & SONS, INC., PUBLICATION

For general information on our other products and services or for technical support, please contact our Customer Care Department within the United States at (800) 762-2974, outside the United States at (317) 572-3993 or fax (317) 572-4002.

Wiley also publishes its books in a variety of electronic formats. Some content that appears in print may not be available in electronic format. For information about Wiley products, visit our web site at www.wiley.com.

Library of Congress Cataloging-in-Publication Data is available.

ISBN 978-0-470-40101-9

10 9 8 7 6 5 4 3 2

CONTENTS

PREFACE

The problems in the book are designed to illustrate the methods, ideas, and approaches to analysis described in each chapter. Each chapter has relatively few problems. There are no "math" problems in the sense of having to derive a mathematical solution to a theoretical exercise. As such, the problems do not lend themselves to providing a partial solutions manual for students and a complete solutions manual for instructors. We suggest that instructors supplement the problems in the text with similar questions using data from their own fields and areas of statistical practice.

This solutions manual presents the methods, computer output and discussion that we would use if we had been assigned the problems in the text. In any data analysis exercise one makes choices along the way, for example, which variables to include and how to scale continuous covariates. There is both art and science in a good data analysis and two experienced analysts may arrive at slightly different models, each of which accomplishes the goals of the analysis. Thus in many problems our solution should not be taken as the only possible one. We encourage instructors to consider alternative solutions and models and to discuss their respective strengths and weaknesses with their students.

We performed most of the calculations in this solutions manual using STATA® (version 10.0). In a few instances SUDAAN® was used. The code presented in the manual is what we used to get the job done and likely does not represent the most elegant or efficient coding. We have made no attempt to use all the "latest" features in the software. In addition, we have no plans to revise the solutions manual to illustrate future software developments. Some of the calculations performed in STATA® could be performed by other statistical packages if they include survey analysis capabilities.

We have made every attempt to make the solutions as accurate as possible. There is a formidable amount of numerical computation and calculation in the manual and there are likely a few errors we missed. We would appreciate learning of these. We do not, however, have the time to react to and comment on alternative solutions to the problems.

As noted in the Preface of the text all data sets may be found at the Wiley ftp site, ftp://ftp.wiley.com/public/sci_tech_med/populations.

Throughout the years we have spent teaching sampling courses using this text, there have been many outstanding students who have struggled with the exercises. We would particularly like to single out Annette Bucher for the careful work she did as her solutions provided us with a model for many of the solutions to be found in this manual.

PAUL S. LEVY
STANLEY LEMESHOW
ERINN M. HADE
AMY K. FERKETICH

Chapter One – Solutions

1.1   *Means, proportions, and totals are examples of:*
    a.   *Summary statistics*
    b.   *Sample persons*
    c.   *Survey reports*
    d.   *Database elements*

Solution: a: Summary statistics

1.2   Sample surveys are least concerned with:
    a.   Production of summary statistics
    b.   *Production of valid and reliable estimates*
    c.   *Describing characteristics of the population*
    d.   *Testing hypotheses*

Solution: d: Testing hypotheses

1.3   *Which of the following is most correct concerning what is included in the sample design?*
    a.   *The sampling plan and statistical reports*
    b.   *The sampling plan and estimation procedures*
    c.   *The sampling plan and cost estimates*
    d.   *The estimation procedures and quality control measures*

Solution: b: The sampling plan and estimation procedures

1.4   *Sample surveys belong to a larger class of studies called:*
    a.   *Cohort studies*
    b.   *Observational studies*
    c.   *Case-control studies*
    d.   *Quasi experiments*

Solution: b: Observational studies

1.5   *Which of the following best describes estimates obtained from a census?*
   a.   *Both sampling and measurement errors present*
   b.   *Sampling but not measurement errors present*
   c.   *Measurement errors but not sampling errors present*
   d.   *Neither sampling nor measurement errors present*

Solution: c: Measurement errors but not sampling errors present

1.6   *Feedback from a pilot study will generally yield which of the following benefits?*
   a.   *Lowering of measurement errors*
   b.   *Lowering of sampling errors*
   c.   *Decrease in costs*
   d.   *All of the above*

Solution: d: All of the above. This is true because a pilot survey (if well done) can result in reduced sampling errors and reduced costs as well as in lowered measurement errors. However, it should be noted that this answer doesn't agree with the one in the back of the text. There we said (a): Lowering of measurement errors since, traditionally, the focus of pilot surveys has been to sharpen up the survey instruments which results, primarily, in reduced sampling errors.

1.7   *You are the chief executive officer of a hospital and wish to know within a very short time the proportion covered by third-party carriers other than Medicare or Medicaid of all inpatient admissions within 2006. How would you go about determining this proportion?*

Solution: Take a sample of patient records from the entire pool of 2006 hospital records. Record the type of insurance the patient had and use the sample proportion as an estimate of the population proportion.

1.8   *As the same CEO as in Exercise 1.7, you wish to estimate the mean out-of-pocket costs per inpatient admission. How could you go about determining this?*

Solution: Using the same sample of patient records, note the out-of-pocket costs for each patient. Use the sample mean as an estimate of the population mean cost.

Chapter Two – Solutions

2.1. *The accompanying table presents a population of five hospitals denoted by A, B, C, D, and E. The total number of beds is given for each hospital.*

Hospital	Number of Beds
A	160
B	220
C	850
D	510
E	110

Solution: Construct a STATA data file consisting of 5 records and two variables (hospital and number of beds). (You can enter the data using the data editor.)

```
. list
       Hospital       Beds
  1.          A        160
  2.          B        220
  3.          C        850
  4.          D        510
  5.          E        110
```

a. *Compute the mean number of beds and the standard deviation of the distribution of the number of beds in the population of five hospitals.*

Solution:

```
. sum Beds, detail
                            Beds
-------------------------------------------------------------
        Percentiles      Smallest
 1%         110             110
 5%         110             160
10%         110             220      Obs                    5
25%         160             510      Sum of Wgt.            5

50%         220                      Mean                 370
                          Largest    Std. Dev.       309.9193
75%         510             160
90%         850             220      Variance           96050
95%         850             510      Skewness        .7805045
99%         850             850      Kurtosis        2.048956
```

```
. display sqrt((96050*4) / 5)
277.20029
```

The population mean number of beds is 370 and the standard deviation of the distribution of the number of beds in the population is 277.2003.

b. *How many samples of two hospitals can be drawn from this population of five hospitals?*

Solution: Assuming a simple random sample design, the number of possible samples is 5 choose 2, or 10.

c. *List each of the possible samples of two hospitals and compute the mean number of beds per hospital for each sample.*

Solution: Construct a file giving each sample and its value.

```
. list

        sample1    sample2       x1         x2
  1.          A          B       160        220
  2.          A          C       160        850
  3.          A          D       160        510
  4.          A          E       160        110
  5.          B          C       220        850
  6.          B          D       220        510
  7.          B          E       220        110
  8.          C          D       850        510
  9.          C          E       850        110
 10.          D          E       510        110

. gen xbar=(x1+x2)/2

. list xbar

        xbar
  1.       190
  2.       505
  3.       335
  4.       135
  5.       535
  6.       365
  7.       165
  8.       680
  9.       480
 10.       310
```

d. *Assuming each of the samples listed in part (c) is equally likely, compute the mean and variance of the distribution of sample means. How does the mean of this distribution compare with the population mean?*

Solution:

```
. sum xbar, detail

                              xbar
-------------------------------------------------------------
      Percentiles      Smallest
 1%         135              135
 5%         135              165
10%         150              190      Obs                 10
25%         190              310      Sum of Wgt.         10

50%         350                       Mean               370
                        Largest       Std. Dev.      178.932
75%         505              480
90%       607.5              505       Variance      32016.67
95%         680              535       Skewness     .2124264
99%         680              680       Kurtosis     1.967362


. display 32016.67 * 9 / 10
28815.003
```

The mean of the sampling distribution, 370, is equal to the population mean. The variance is equal to 28,815.

e. *Calculate the standard error of the mean. How does this value compare with the population standard deviation?*

Solution:

```
. display sqrt(32016.67 * 9 / 10)
169.74982
```

The standard error of the mean is 169.75, and this is less than the population standard deviation which is 277.20.

f. How many different samples of four hospitals can be drawn from this population? List each of these samples plus the sample mean for each sample.

Solution: The number of samples of 4 hospitals from the population of 5 hospitals is equal to the number of combinations of 5 objects, 4 at a time and is equal to 5. To list these, construct a STATA data file consisting of 5 records with the values for number of beds in each sample hospital:

```
. gen xbar = (x1+x2+x3+x4) / 4

. list

        Sample      x1       x2       x3       x4       xbar
   1.    ABCD       160      220      850      510      435
   2.    ABCE       160      220      850      110      335
   3.    ABDE       160      220      510      110      250
   4.    ACDE       160      850      510      110      407.5
   5.    BCDE       220      850      510      110      422.5
```

g. Calculate the mean and variance for the sample means listed in part (f). How do these compare with the mean and variance obtained in part (d)?

Solution:

```
. sum xbar, detail

                              xbar
-------------------------------------------------------------
      Percentiles      Smallest
 1%       250             250
 5%       250             335
10%       250             407.5      Obs                    5
25%       335             422.5      Sum of Wgt.            5

50%       407.5                      Mean                 370
                         Largest     Std. Dev.        77.47984
75%       422.5            335
90%       435             407.5      Variance         6003.125
95%       435             422.5      Skewness        -.7805045
99%       435             435        Kurtosis         2.048956


. display (6003.125 * 4) / 5
4802.5
```

The mean of the sampling distribution is 370, which is equal to the population mean and the mean obtained in part (d). The variance is 4802.5, and this value is smaller than the variance obtained in part (d), 28,815.

2.2.   *For each of the following problems indicate how you would carry out a sample and specify these entities:*

   a.   *Population*
   b.   *The variable(s)*
   c.   *The elementary unit*
   d.   *The frame*
   e.   *The enumeration unit*

   1.   *Suppose we wish to estimate the average cost of an appendectomy in a certain state. There are 27 hospitals in this state.*

      a.   The population includes all of the patients who had an appendectomy in that state, in a specified period of time.
      b.   The variable of interest is the cost associated with the appendectomy.
      c.   The elementary unit is the patient who received the surgery.
      d.   The frame is the list of patients who had an appendectomy during a specified period of time. There will be one list from each hospital.
      e.   The enumeration unit is the patient who had the surgery.

   2.   *Suppose we wish to do a nutritional survey in order to estimate the average amount of fiber consumed by individuals in a certain city. Suppose there is no list of families available for the city but there is a map of the city showing each block in detail.*

      a.   The population consists of all individuals who live in that city during a specified period of time.
      b.   The variable of interest is the amount of fiber consumed.
      c.   The elementary unit is the individual person.
      d.   The frame is the list of city blocks.
      e.   The enumeration unit is the household.

   3.   *Suppose we are interested in the proportion of calves that die prior to the first year of life at all dairy farms in a particular state.*

      a.   The population consists of all calves born at dairy farms at least one year ago in that particular state. The time period will have to be specified, for example, from one year ago to two years ago.
      b.   The variable of interest is whether or not the calf died during the first year of life.
      c.   The elementary unit is the individual calf.
      d.   The frame is the list of dairy farms.
      e.   The enumeration unit is the calf.

2.3.   *Suppose that a survey is being planned for purposes of estimating the average number of hours spent exercising daily by adults (18 years of age or older) living in a certain community. A list of all individuals living in the town is not available; however, a list of all households is available at the office of the town clerk. For simplicity, suppose this list consists of nine households and that the information you would collect, were you to visit each household, is as shown in the accompanying table.*

Household	Number of adults	Aggregate Number of Hours Spent Exercising by All Adults
1	2	1
2	3	3
3	2	7
4	5	8
5	3	4
6	1	0
7	2	1
8	3	2
9	2	0

a. *Define these:*
   1. *Population*
   2. *Elementary unit*
   3. *Enumeration unit*
   4. *Frame*
   5. *Variable*

   Solution:
   1.   The population is the totality of all adults living in the community.
   2.   The elementary unit is the individual adult in the community.
   3.   The enumeration unit is the household.
   4.   The frame is the list of households.
   5.   The variable is the number of hours spent exercising.

b. *Devise a sampling plan to estimate the average daily time expenditure on exercising by adults living in the community.*

   Solution:
   Take a sample of households. Within each sampled household, ask each adult household member the question on hours spent exercising.

c. Select all samples of two households from this frame and compute the average exercising time per person for each sample.

Solution: Construct a STATA data file consisting of 36 records with the values for number of adults and the aggregate number of hours spent exercising in each sample household.

```
. list

        Sample  Adults_1  Adults_2  Exerhr_1  Exerhr_2
 1.       12        2         3         1         3
 2.       13        2         2         1         7
 3.       14        2         5         1         8
 4.       15        2         3         1         4
 5.       16        2         1         1         0
 6.       17        2         2         1         1
 7.       18        2         3         1         2
 8.       19        2         2         1         0
 9.       23        3         2         3         7
10.       24        3         5         3         8
11.       25        3         3         3         4
12.       26        3         1         3         0
13.       27        3         2         3         1
14.       28        3         3         3         2
15.       29        3         2         3         0
16.       34        2         5         7         8
17.       35        2         3         7         4
18.       36        2         1         7         0
19.       37        2         2         7         1
20.       38        2         3         7         2
21.       39        2         2         7         0
22.       45        5         3         8         4
23.       46        5         1         8         0
24.       47        5         2         8         1
25.       48        5         3         8         2
26.       49        5         2         8         0
27.       56        3         1         4         0
28.       57        3         2         4         1
29.       58        3         3         4         2
30.       59        3         2         4         0
31.       67        1         2         0         1
32.       68        1         3         0         2
33.       69        1         2         0         0
34.       78        2         3         1         2
35.       79        2         2         1         0
36.       89        3         2         2         0
```

Next, compute the average exercise time per person for each sample.

```
. gen adults = (Adults_1+ Adults_2)/2

. gen exerhour = (Exerhr_1+ Exerhr_2) / 2

. gen exhr_ad = exerhour / adults
```

d. Compute the expected value of your estimate and compare this to the actual population parameter.

Solution:

```
. list exhr_ad

        exhr_ad
  1.         .8
  2.          2
  3.   1.285714
  4.          1
  5.  .3333333
  6.         .5
  7.         .6
  8.        .25
  9.          2
 10.      1.375
 11.   1.166667
 12.        .75
 13.         .8
 14.  .8333333
 15.         .6
 16.   2.142857
 17.        2.2
 18.   2.333333
 19.          2
 20.        1.8
 21.       1.75
 22.        1.5
 23.   1.333333
 24.   1.285714
 25.       1.25
 26.   1.142857
 27.          1
 28.          1
 29.          1
 30.         .8
 31.  .3333333
 32.         .5
 33.          0
 34.         .6
 35.        .25
 36.         .4
```

```
. sum exhr_ad, detail

                              exhr_ad
-------------------------------------------------------------
      Percentiles      Smallest
 1%           0               0
 5%         .25             .25
10%    .3333333             .25        Obs                36
25%          .6        .3333333        Sum of Wgt.        36

50%           1                        Mean         1.080985
                        Largest        Std. Dev.     .6286071
75%      1.4375               2
90%           2        2.142857        Variance      .3951469
95%         2.2             2.2        Skewness      .3840009
99%    2.333333        2.333333        Kurtosis      2.171174

. display sqrt((0.3951469 * 35) / 36)
0.61981497
```

The mean of the sampling distribution of exhr_ad is 1.0810, which is not equal to 1.1304, the population mean.

e. *Calculate the standard error of your estimate.*

   Solution: The standard error of exhr_ad is 0.6198.

2.4. *As part of an AIDS education program, 120 intravenous drug users seronegative for HIV (Human Immunodeficiency Virus) at a first screening were given instructions on sterilizing their needles with bleach and practicing "safe sex." One year after the program's inception, a sample of 30 of these subjects was taken by numbering the participants from 1 to 120 and taking all subjects whose numbers are divisible by 4 (e.g., 4, 8, 12, etc.).*

a. *What is the chance of each individual being chosen in the sample?*

   Solution: The chance of selection is 1 for the 30 persons whose numbers are divisible by 4 and 0 for all others. If we assume that the numbering is totally random then we can say that the chance of selection is 30/120 or 0.25 for each person.

b. *If subjects 1, 3, 4, 8, 29, and 65 are seropositive for HIV, what is the proportion of seroconverted subjects for this population?*

   Solution: Population proportion is 6/120=0.05

c. *What is the proportion of seroconverted subjects in the sample? Is this an unbiased estimate of the population proportion?*

   Solution: Sample proportion is 2/30 =0.067. This is an unbiased estimate if we assume that a random start was taken.

2.5. As part of a marketing program, a city block containing 4 households was selected and a sample of 3 households was sampled as follows: Jeremiah, the research assistant, identified the households and numbered each household from 1 to 4. He then was to list all combinations of the 4 households 2 at a time. These are:

1 and 2	1 and 3	1 and 4
2 and 3	2 and 4	3 and 4

Unfortunately, Jeremiah got this job because he was related to the Department Chairman, and he was very careless. He forgot the combination 3 and 4. He chose a random number between 1 and 5 (it turned out to be 4) which corresponded to the combination 2 and 3. Thus households 2 and 3 were sampled. The variable of interest was out-of-pocket medical expenses incurred by the household. These were as follows for the 4 households

Household	Expenses ($)
1	345.00
2	126.00
3	492.00
4	962.00

a. Based on Jeremiah's sampling procedure, what is the mean, standard error, and MSE of the estimated mean out-of-pocket medical expenses?

Solution: Construct a STATA data file consisting of 5 records (sample with 3 and 4 is not included) with the values for out-of-pocket expenses in each sample household:

```
. gen xbar = (Expense1 + Expense2) / 2

. list

        Sample  Expense1  Expense2     xbar
  1.        12       345       126    235.5
  2.        13       345       492    418.5
  3.        14       345       962    653.5
  4.        23       126       492      309
  5.        24       126       962      544
```

```
. sum xbar, detail

                              xbar
-------------------------------------------------------------
        Percentiles      Smallest
 1%        235.5           235.5
 5%        235.5           309
10%        235.5           418.5        Obs                 5
25%        309             544          Sum of Wgt.         5

50%        418.5                        Mean            432.1
                          Largest       Std. Dev.    169.9483
75%        544             309
90%        653.5           418.5        Variance     28882.43
95%        653.5           544          Skewness     .1586973
99%        653.5           653.5        Kurtosis     1.604527

. display (28882.43 * 4) / 5
23105.944

. display sqrt((28882.43 * 4) / 5)
152.00639

. display (345+126+492+962)/4
481.25

. display 23105.944 + (481.25-432.1)^2
25521.666
```

The mean is equal to 432.1, the variance is 23,105.9, and the standard error is 152.01. The mean square error is equal to 25,521.67.

(a) *Is the estimate derived from this sampling procedure unbiased?*

```
. display (345 + 126 + 492 + 962) /
    4
481.25
```

The population mean is equal to 481.25, which is greater than that obtained using Jeremiah's procedure.

b. *Does every household have the same chance of appearing in the sample? Why or why not?*

Solution: Households 1 and 2 appear in 60% of the samples, while households 3 and 4 appear in only 40% of the samples. So, no, every household does not have the same chance of appearing in the sample.

2.6.   *It is desired to perform a quality control audit of laboratory data from a large clinical trial for purposes of estimating the proportion of laboratory values in the database that are invalid. There are 394 patients in the clinical trial, and each person has had from 60 to 200 laboratory determinations during the course of the trial. The sampling plan chosen was to select a random sample of 10 patients and for each sample person take a random sample of 10 laboratory determinations, which would then be checked against the patient medical record for accuracy.*

a.   *What are the elementary units in this sample design?*

    Solution: The elementary units are the laboratory determinations.

b.   *What are the sampling units in this sample design?*

    Solution: The sampling units are the persons.

c.   *Does each person in the population have an equal chance of being selected in the sample?*

    Solution: Each person has an equal chance of being selected in the sample

d.   *Does each laboratory determination in the population have an equal chance of being selected in the sample?*

    Solution: Each laboratory determination does not have an equal chance of being selected. The probability of a laboratory determination being selected is the product of the probability of a person being selected ($=10/394$) and the probability of a particular laboratory determination from that person is chosen, given that the person was chosen ($=10/n_i$, where n_i is the number of laboratory determinations done on the patient). Clearly this is not the same for each person.

2.7.   *Data from the sample described in Exercise 2.6 are shown below:*

Subject	Total Invalid Laboratory Values in 10 Sampled
1	1
2	0
3	2
4	0
5	1
6	0
7	0
8	0
9	0
10	1

Based on these data, what is the estimated proportion of laboratory results that are invalid?

Solution: Construct a STATA data file consisting of 10 records with the values for number of invalid laboratory values for each sampled subject (you can enter the data using the data editor):

```
. gen propinvd = Invalid / 10

. list

        Subject   Invalid   propinvd
  1.        1        1         .1
  2.        2        0          0
  3.        3        2         .2
  4.        4        0          0
  5.        5        1         .1
  6.        6        0          0
  7.        7        0          0
  8.        8        0          0
  9.        9        0          0
 10.       10        1         .1
```

Next, use the sum procedure in STATA to obtain the correct estimate of the proportion of invalid results.

```
. sum propinvd

    Variable |      Obs        Mean    Std. Dev.       Min        Max
-------------+--------------------------------------------------------
    propinvd |       10         .05    .0707107          0         .2
```

The estimated proportion of laboratory results that are invalid is 0.05. Note that the more correct procedure would be to use the svymean command discussed in Chapter 3. This would give the same estimate of the mean but a more correct estimate of the standard error of the mean. We do not propose this here because concepts of simple random sampling are not introduced until Chapter 3.

2.8. *The following table shows the total number of laboratory determinations for the 10 sample patients described in Exercise 2.6 as well as the number of invalid determinations among the 10 determinations sampled:*

Subject	Total Laboratory Values	Total Invalid Laboratory Values in 10 Sampled
1	103	1
2	123	0
3	93	2
4	200	0
5	128	1
6	165	0
7	132	0
8	189	0
9	176	0
10	180	1

Solution:

```
. list

       Subject    Invalid    propinvd    Totalval
 1.        1          1          .1         103
 2.        2          0           0         123
 3.        3          2          .2          93
 4.        4          0           0         200
 5.        5          1          .1         128
 6.        6          0           0         165
 7.        7          0           0         132
 8.        8          0           0         189
 9.        9          0           0         176
10.       10          1          .1         180
```

Use the summation command in STATA with the frequency weights option to obtain the correct estimate of the proportion of invalid results.

```
. sum propinvd [fweight=Totalval]

    Variable |      Obs        Mean    Std. Dev.        Min         Max
-------------+-----------------------------------------------------------
    propinvd |     1489     .040094    .0604441           0          .2
```

The estimated proportion of laboratory results that are invalid, using all of the data, is 0.04 which differs substantially from the value of 0.05 found when all of the data were not used.

2.9. *Match the term in column 1 with the most appropriate term in column 2.*

Column 1	Column 2
1. MSE	A. $\sum_{i=1} x_i$
2. Reliability	B. Population
3. Bias	C. Accuracy
4. Universe	D. $\sum_{i=1} X_i$
5. Sample Total	E. Validity
6. Population Total	F. Variance

1.	C
2.	F
3.	E
4.	B
5.	A
6.	D

Chapter Three – Solutions

3.1   *From the data in Table 2.1, using simple random sampling, take ten different samples of six physicians. For each sample compute approximate 95% confidence intervals for the average number of household visits per physician. For how many of these calculated 95% confidence intervals is the true population mean within the boundaries of the intervals? If this number is much higher or lower than expected, how do you explain it? (Start with the first random number in the upper left-hand corner of Table A.1 in the Appendix and read down the columns, going no further than row 35.)*

Solution: The following samples are included in this problem.

Sample	Physicians	Number of Visits
1	10, 22, 24, 09, 07, 02	22, 0, 1, 0, 12, 0
2	01, 07, 02, 05, 25, 09	5, 12, 0, 7, 0, 0
3	05, 06, 14, 12, 21, 20	7, 0, 4, 5, 8, 0
4	04, 01, 25, 22, 06, 11	4, 5, 0, 0, 0, 0
5	05, 22, 04, 25, 02, 16	7, 0, 4, 0, 0, 0
6	07, 10, 03, 08, 09, 14	12, 22, 1, 0, 0, 4
7	24, 07, 12, 06, 18, 17	1, 12, 5, 0, 0, 7
8	23, 09, 13, 19, 24, 18	0, 0, 6, 37, 1, 0
9	16, 20, 18, 13, 19, 04	0, 0, 0, 6, 37, 4
10	14, 06, 25, 20, 18, 15	4, 0, 0, 0, 0, 8

Using STATA:

```
. gen N = 25

. gen wt = N / 6

. svyset _n [pweight=wt], fpc(N)

      pweight: wt
          VCE: linearized
  Single unit: missing
     Strata 1: <one>
         SU 1: <observations>
        FPC 1: N

. svy: mean  S1 S2 S3 S4 S5 S6 S7 S8 S9 S10
(running mean on estimation sample)

Survey: Mean estimation

Number of strata =        1      Number of obs    =        6
Number of PSUs   =        6      Population size  =       25
                                 Design df        =        5


-----------------------------------------------------------------
             |               Linearized
             |       Mean    Std. Err.    [95% Conf. Interval]
-------------+---------------------------------------------------
         S1  |   5.833333     3.280616     -2.59976     14.26643
         S2  |          4     1.758029    -.5191579     8.519158
         S3  |          4     1.212161      .884042     7.115958
         S4  |        1.5     .8346656    -.6455762     3.645576
         S5  |   1.833333     1.065729    -.9062096     4.572876
         S6  |        6.5     3.149286    -1.595496      14.5955
         S7  |   4.166667     1.705612    -.2177477     8.551081
         S8  |   7.333333     5.238745    -6.133288     20.79995
         S9  |   7.833333     5.164473    -5.442366     21.10903
        S10  |          2     1.191078    -1.061763     5.061763
-----------------------------------------------------------------
```

The true population mean is 5.08 visits (from page 17 in text). In the above table, 7 of the 10 approximate confidence intervals contain the true population mean, or 70% of the samples. This is lower than expected because 9 or all 10 of the 95% confidence intervals should contain the population mean. The samples that have intervals that do not cover the true mean are ones that contain 4 zeroes, or 66.7% of the sample. In the population, only 44% of the observations are zero, which is much lower than 66.7%. Thus, the samples are unusual with respect to the proportion of zeroes contained in them.

Note: The confidence intervals reported here are slightly different from those in the back of the book. STATA uses the t distribution when it computes the intervals, rather than the standard normal distribution. Also, for the intervals with a lower bound less than zero, the lower bound should be set to zero.

3.2   *How many simple random samples of 15 elements can be taken from a population containing 65 elements?*

Solution: Assuming a simple random sample design, the number of possible samples is 65 choose 15, or $2.073746998 \times 10^{14}$.

3.3   *From the data in Table 3.8 estimate the proportion of all workers in the plant having an fvc less than 70% of that expected on the basis of age, sex, and height. Give a 95% confidence interval for this estimated proportion.*

Solution: Use the workers.dta file on the ftp site.

```
. list
        worker      exposure           fvc        popsize          wt1
  1.        22            1            64           1200            30
  2.        21            2            70           1200            30
  3.        31            3            84           1200            30
  4.         7            1            82           1200            30
  5.        20            2            99           1200            30
  6.        33            3            89           1200            30
  7.         1            3            81           1200            30
  8.         8            1            99           1200            30
  9.        11            1            71           1200            30
 10.        24            2            72           1200            30
 11.        15            3            77           1200            30
 12.        26            3            96           1200            30
 13.        17            3            62           1200            30
 14.        12            3            88           1200            30
 15.        30            1            87           1200            30
 16.        13            2            84           1200            30
 17.        25            3            95           1200            30
 18.        27            3            62           1200            30
 19.        28            3            67           1200            30
 20.        19            3            91           1200            30
 21.        38            3            98           1200            30
 22.         4            2            91           1200            30
 23.         2            3            64           1200            30
 24.        18            3            67           1200            30
 25.        37            3            80           1200            30
 26.         3            2            85           1200            30
 27.        34            3            65           1200            30
 28.         5            3            60           1200            30
 29.        29            3            95           1200            30
 30.        35            3            67           1200            30
 31.        36            3            69           1200            30
 32.        39            3            65           1200            30
 33.        16            3            76           1200            30
 34.         9            3            96           1200            30
 35.        10            3            91           1200            30
 36.         6            1            97           1200            30
 37.        14            3            85           1200            30
 38.        40            3            84           1200            30
 39.        32            3            89           1200            30
 40.        23            3            72           1200            30
```

```
. svyset _n [pweight=wt1], fpc(popsize)

        pweight: wt1
            VCE: linearized
    Single unit: missing
```

```
      Strata 1: <one>
         SU 1: <observations>
        FPC 1: popsize


. gen fvclt70=(fvc<70)

. tab fvclt70

    fvclt70 |      Freq.      Percent        Cum.
------------+-----------------------------------
          0 |        29        72.50       72.50
          1 |        11        27.50      100.00
------------+-----------------------------------
      Total |        40       100.00

. svy: mean fvclt70
(running mean on estimation sample)

Survey: Mean estimation

Number of strata =          1      Number of obs     =        40
Number of PSUs   =         40      Population size   =      1200
                                   Design df         =        39


-----------------------------------------------------------------
            |             Linearized
            |    Mean     Std. Err.      [95% Conf. Interval]
------------+----------------------------------------------------
    fvclt70 |    .275     .0702977      .1328094     .4171906
-----------------------------------------------------------------
```

The estimated proportion of all workers in the plant having an fvc is less than 70% of that expected is 0.275. A 95% confidence interval for this estimate is 0.13 to 0.42.

3.4   *From the data in Table 3.8 on the workers having low or medium exposure to pulmonary stressors, estimate the proportion who have an fvc below 90% of that expected on the basis of age, sex and height. Give a 95% confidence interval for this proportion.*

Solution: We can perform this calculation in STATA, using the svy: mean command. First, create an indicator variable that takes on the value of 1 if the fvc is below 90 and 0 if it is greater than equal to 90. Next, create another indicator variable that takes on the value of 1 if the worker has a low or medium exposure to pulmonary stressors and 0 if the exposure is high. Then perform the svy: mean procedure in STATA with the *over* command.

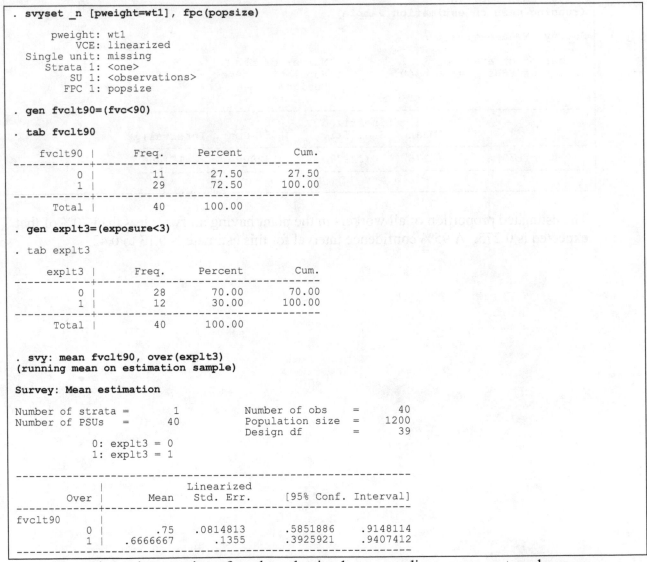

```
. svyset _n [pweight=wt1], fpc(popsize)

      pweight: wt1
          VCE: linearized
  Single unit: missing
    Strata 1: <one>
        SU 1: <observations>
       FPC 1: popsize

. gen fvclt90=(fvc<90)

. tab fvclt90

   fvclt90 |      Freq.     Percent        Cum.
-----------+-----------------------------------
         0 |         11       27.50       27.50
         1 |         29       72.50      100.00
-----------+-----------------------------------
     Total |         40      100.00

. gen explt3=(exposure<3)

. tab explt3

   explt3 |      Freq.     Percent        Cum.
-----------+-----------------------------------
         0 |         28       70.00       70.00
         1 |         12       30.00      100.00
-----------+-----------------------------------
     Total |         40      100.00


. svy: mean fvclt90, over(explt3)
(running mean on estimation sample)

Survey: Mean estimation

Number of strata =        1        Number of obs    =       40
Number of PSUs   =       40        Population size  =     1200
                                   Design df        =       39

            0: explt3 = 0
            1: explt3 = 1

-----------------------------------------------------------------
            |             Linearized
       Over |      Mean    Std. Err.     [95% Conf. Interval]
------------+----------------------------------------------------
fvclt90     |
          0 |       .75    .0814813     .5851886    .9148114
          1 | .6666667       .1355     .3925921    .9407412
-----------------------------------------------------------------
```

The estimated proportion of workers, having low or medium exposure to pulmonary stressors, who have an FVC below 90% of that expected, is 0.67. A 95% confidence interval for that estimate is 0.39 to 0.94.

3.5   *From the data in Table 3.8, estimate the proportion of workers in the plant having low or medium exposure to pulmonary stressors. Give a 95% confidence interval for this estimated proportion.*

```
. gen lowmed=(exposure != 3)

. tab lowmed

     lowmed |      Freq.      Percent        Cum.
------------+-----------------------------------
          0 |         28        70.00       70.00
          1 |         12        30.00      100.00
------------+-----------------------------------
      Total |         40       100.00

. svy: mean lowmed
(running mean on estimation sample)

Survey: Mean estimation

Number of strata =          1        Number of obs    =        40
Number of PSUs   =         40        Population size  =      1200
                                     Design df        =        39


------------------------------------------------------------------
            |              Linearized
            |     Mean     Std. Err.      [95% Conf. Interval]
------------+-----------------------------------------------------
     lowmed |       .3     .0721466       .1540698      .4459302
------------------------------------------------------------------
```

Solution: The estimated proportion of workers in the plant having low or medium exposure to pulmonary stressors is 0.30. A 95% confidence interval for this estimate is 0.15 to 0.45.

3.6   *A survey of workers is to be taken in a large plant that makes products similar to those made in the plant from which the data in Table 3.8 are obtained. The purposes of the survey are to estimate (a) the proportion of all workers having an fvc below 70% and (b) the mean fvc among all workers. Estimates are needed within 5% of the true value of the parameter being estimated. How large a sample of workers is required? The plant employs 5000 workers.*

Solution: $N = 5000$, $\varepsilon = 0.05$; Let $\alpha = 0.05$, $z = 1.96$

From Box 3.5, relation 3.16:

Virtual Certainty:

```
. display (3^2 * 5000 * 0.275 * 0.725) / ((4999 * 0.05^2 * 0.275^2) + (3^2 * 0.275
    * 0.725))
3275.0064
```

95% Confidence:

```
. display (1.96^2 * 5000 * 0.275 * 0.725) / ((4999 * 0.05^2 * 0.275^2) + (1.96^2 *
    0.275 * 0.725))
2238.1648
```

The required sample size is 3275.01 or 3276 for virtual certainty, and 2238.17 or 2239 persons for 95% confidence.

3.7   *A community within a city contains 3000 households and 10,000 persons. For purposes of planning a community satellite to the local health department, it is desired to estimate the total number of physician visits made during a calendar year by members of the community. For this information to be useful, it should be accurate to within 10% of the true value. A small pilot survey of 10 households, conducted for purposes of gathering preliminary information, yielded the accompanying data on physician visits made during the previous calendar year. Using these data as preliminary information, determine the sample size needed to meet the specifications of the survey.*

Household	No. of Persons in Household	No. of Physician Visits Per Person During Previous Year
1	3	4.0
2	6	4.5
3	2	8.0
4	5	3.4
5	2	0.5
6	3	7.0
7	4	8.5
8	2	6.0
9	6	4.0
10	4	7.5

Solution: $N = 3000$, $\varepsilon = 0.10$; Let $\alpha = 0.05$, $z = 1.96$

From Box 3.5, relation 3.16:

```
. gen tot_vis = Persons*Mdvisits

. sum tot_vis

    Variable |      Obs       Mean   Std. Dev.         Min        Max
-------------+-------------------------------------------------------
     tot_vis |       10       19.4   9.845473           1         34

. display ((2999 / 3000) * 9.84573^2) / 19.4^2
.25748243
```

Virtual Certainty:

```
. display (3^2 * 3000 * 0.2575) / ((3^2 * 0.2575) + (2999 * 0.10^2))
215.19771
```

95% Confidence:

```
. display (1.96^2 * 3000 * 0.2575) / ((1.96^2 * 0.2575) + (2999 * 0.10^2))
95.794431
```

The required sample size for virtual certainty is 215.2 or 216 and for 95% confidence, the sample size should be 95.8 or 96 households.

3.8 A section of a random number table is reproduced here:

06	97	37	77
08	00	39	81
14	08	58	01
22	17	24	19
75	73	12	79
69	59	32	53
54	03	48	44

a. Starting with the first random number in the upper left-hand corner of this table and reading down the columns, select a sample of 6 of the 25 physicians listed in Table 2.1.

Solution: reading down the columns, select the first six unique numbers that are between 1 and 25. The following physicians will be included in the sample.

Physician	No. of Visits
06	0
08	0
14	4
22	0
17	7
03	1

b. Estimate the mean number of household visits made by physicians in the population, and construct a 90% confidence interval for the mean.

```
. gen N=25

. gen wt=25/6

. svyset _n [pweight=wt], fpc(N)

      pweight: wt
          VCE: linearized
  Single unit: missing
     Strata 1: <one>
        SU 1: <observations>
       FPC 1: N

. svy: mean visits, level(90)
(running mean on estimation sample)

Survey: Mean estimation

Number of strata =        1       Number of obs   =        6
Number of PSUs   =        6       Population size =       25
                                  Design df       =        5
--------------------------------------------------------------
             |            Linearized
             |    Mean    Std. Err.     [90% Conf. Interval]
-------------+------------------------------------------------
      visits |      2    1.031504       -.07853    4.07853
--------------------------------------------------------------
```

Solution: The mean number of household visits made by physicians in the population is estimated to be 1.03. A 90% confidence interval for this estimate is 0 to 4.08.

c.   *Estimate the total number X of household visits made by the physicians in the population and construct a 95% confidence interval for X. How does this confidence interval compare to the one given in the Illustrative Example in Section 3.5?*

```
. svy: total visits
(running total on estimation sample)

Survey: Total estimation

Number of strata =        1        Number of obs     =        6
Number of PSUs   =        6        Population size   =       25
                                   Design df         =        5


-----------------------------------------------------------------
                 |              Linearized
                 |     Total    Std. Err.     [95% Conf. Interval]
-----------------+-----------------------------------------------
          visits |        50    25.78759     -16.28912    116.2891
-----------------------------------------------------------------
```

Solution: The total number of household visits made by physicians in the population is estimated to be 50. A 95% confidence interval for this estimate is 0 to 116.3. This estimate is different from the one obtained in Section 3.5. In the sample selected here, 3 of the 6 physicians reported zero visits whereas in the example only one physician reported zero visits. That resulted in a larger estimate of the total and a confidence interval that is far from zero.

d.   *Estimate with virtual certainty, the proportion of physicians in the population making two or more household visits per year.*

```
. gen twovisit=(visits>=2)

. tab twovisit

    twovisit |      Freq.     Percent        Cum.
-------------+-----------------------------------
           0 |          4       66.67       66.67
           1 |          2       33.33      100.00
-------------+-----------------------------------
       Total |          6      100.00

. svy: mean twovisit, level(90)
(running mean on estimation sample)

Survey: Mean estimation

Number of strata =        1        Number of obs     =        6
Number of PSUs   =        6        Population size   =       25
                                   Design df         =        5


-----------------------------------------------------------------
                 |              Linearized
                 |      Mean    Std. Err.     [90% Conf. Interval]
-------------+---------------------------------------------------
    twovisit |   .3333333    .1837873      -.037007    .7036737
-----------------------------------------------------------------
```

Solution: The estimated proportion of physicians in the population making two or more household visits per year is 0.33. A confidence with "virtual certainty" for this estimate is 0 to 1.0.

3.9   *A community in the San Francisco Bay area consists of approximately 50,000 persons, of whom approximately 40% are Caucasians, 25% are African American, 20% are Hispanic and 15% are Asian. It is desired to estimate in this community, the proportion of persons who are not covered by some form of health insurance. One would like to be 95% certain that this estimate is within 15% of the true proportion, which is believed to lie somewhere between 10% and 20% of the total population. Assuming simple random sampling, how large a sample is needed?*

Solution: $N = 50,000$, $\varepsilon = 0.15$, $z = 1.96$

We need to compute two sample sizes, one assuming the true proportion is 0.10 and the second assuming it is 0.20. The larger of the two calculated sample sizes will be the recommended sample size.

From Box 3.5, relation 3.16:

Low End ($P_y = 0.10$):

```
. display (1.96^2 * 50000 * 0.1 * 0.9) / ((1.96^2 * 0.1 * 0.9) + (49999 *
0.15^2 *0.10^2))

1490.8518
```

High End ($P_y = 0.20$):

```
. display (1.96^2 * 50000 * 0.2 * 0.8) / ((1.96^2 * 0.2 * 0.8) + (49999 *
0.15^2 * 0.20^2))

673.76166
```

The required sample size for this project is 1491 subjects.

3.10 *In the previous example, if a simple random sample of the entire population is to be taken, how large a sample is required in order to be 95% certain of estimating within 10% of the true value, the proportion of the Asian population not covered by some form of health insurance (again assuming that the true value lies between 10% and 20%).*

Solution: We have to calculate a sample size for the Asian population using the specifications given. Then, we divide this number by a 0.15 because we are assuming that 15% of a simple random sample of this community would be Asian.

From Box 3.5, relation 3.16

Low End ($P_y = 0.10$):

```
. display (1.96^2 * 50000 * 0.1 * 0.9) / ((1.96^2 * 0.1 * 0.9) +
(49999 * 0.1^2 * 0.10^2))
3233.8854
```

High End ($P_y = 0.20$):

```
. display (1.96^2 * 50000 * 0.2 * 0.8) / ((1.96^2 * 0.2 * 0.8) +
(49999 * 0.1^2 * 0.20^2))
1490.8518
```

We choose the larger of the two numbers, 3234, for our required sample size of Asians. Now, we divide this number by 0.15, and this results in a total sample size of 21,560 individuals.

3.11 *A city contains 20 neighborhood health clinics and it is desired to take a sample of 5 of these clinics for purposes of estimating the total number of persons from all these clinics who had been given, during the past 12 month period, prescriptions for a recently approved antidepressant drug. If one assumes that the mean number of patients seen at these clinics is 1500 per year with the standard deviation of this distribution among clinics being equal to 300, and that approximately 5% of all patients regardless of clinic are given this drug, is a simple random sample of 5 of these clinics likely to yield an estimate that is within 20% of the true value?*

Solution: First, we have to calculate the number of patients on the drug and the standard deviation of this estimate.

$E(x_i) = 1500(0.05) = 75$, $\sigma_x = 300*(0.05) = 15$

Next, we calculate $V = 15/75 = 0.20$. Finally, $N = 20$, $n = 5$, and $z = 1.96$.

```
. display (1.96^2 * 20 * 0.20^2) / ((1.96^2 * 0.20^2) + (19 * 0.20^2))
3.3636873
```

Since our calculated sample size is 3.36 and this is less than the number of samples that we plan to take, we can conclude that a sample of 5 clinics is adequate.

3.12   *A company containing 700 employees is planning to test employees for working under the influence of illicit drugs (e.g., cannabis, cocaine). During the course of a year, a sample of 3 days will be selected for testing and on each of these days, a simple random sample of 50 employees will be selected to be tested. Employees will not be excluded from being tested on the second or third testing date even if they had been tested on previous occasions. If an employee is always working under the influence of cocaine, what is his/her chance of being detected in this testing program (assume that anyone under the influence of one of the illicit drugs who is sampled and tested will have a positive test for that drug)?*

Solution: Define three events d_1, d_2, and d_3 as the events of being selected into the samples on days 1, 2, and 3, respectively. Then, using probability theory,

$$P(\text{detected}) = 1 - P(\text{not detected on any test})$$
$$= 1 - (1 - P(d_1)) * (1 - P(d_2)) * (1 - P(d_3))$$

The probability of being detected at any one time is 50/700 if we assume that the person is always under the influence and that there are no false negative tests.

```
. display 1-(1 - (50 / 700))^3
.19934402
```

If an employee is under the influence all of the time, the chance of being detected is 19.9%.

3.13   *In the previous exercise, what is the employee's chance of being detected if he/she is "under the influence" on the job only 10% of the time?*

Solution: The solution is very similar to that in 3.12, although the probability of being detected at any one time is now (50/700)*0.10 since the employee is under the influence 10% of the time.

```
. display 1-(1 - (0.10)*(50 / 700))^3
.02127587
```

If an employee is under the influence on the job only 10% of the time, the chance of being detected is 2.1%.

Chapter Four – Solutions

4.1 *Suppose the local Childhood Lead Poisoning Prevention Council in a metropolitan area in western Tennessee undertakes the responsibility of determining the proportion of homes in a certain development of 120 homes with unsafe lead levels. Because of the great expense involved in performing spectrometric testing of interior wall, ceilings, floors, baseboards, cabinets, and other obvious lead hazards such as crib bars, as well as of exterior sidings, porches and porch rails, it was decided to select a sample of the homes under study. A good up-to-date data frame exists for sampling purposes. This frame is a street listing containing the address and owner of each home for each of the streets in the target area. It was decided to select a 1 in 3 sample of homes. Let us assume that the only houses with serious lead hazard problems are the 26th, 27th, 28th, and 29th on the list.*

a. *Suppose the random number 2 was chosen to start the sequence. Estimate the proportion of homes with lead hazards from the sample.*

Solution: $N = 120$, $k = 3$, houses 26, 27, 28, 29 are affected, $n = N/k = 120/3 = 40$

If we start with house 2, we sample homes 2, 5, 8, 11, 14, 17, 20, 23, 26, 29, …

Our estimate of the proportion of homes with lead hazards is:

$$p_y = {}^2/_{40} = 0.05$$

b. *Obtain a 95% confidence interval for the proportion of homes with lead hazards. What assumption did you make?*

Solution: Estimated 95% confidence interval for the proportion:

$$0.05 \pm 1.96 * (0.05 * 0.95/39)^{1/2} * ((120 - 40)/120)^{1/2}$$
$$= 0.05 \pm 1.96 * 0.02849 = 0.05 \pm 0.0559$$

The estimated 95% confidence interval is (0, 0.106).

We assumed here that the list is in random sequence. Thus, the estimate of the standard error was not biased.

c. *What is the true variance of the distribution of the estimated proportion of homes with lead hazards? How does this compare with the variance estimated in part (b)?*

Solution: Three possible values of p_y are $1/40 = 0.025$, $2/40 = 0.05$, and $1/40 = 0.025$.

$$E(p_y) = \left(\frac{1}{3}\right) * (0.025 + 0.05 + 0.025) = 0.0333$$

$$Var(p_y) = \sum (p_y - E(p_y))^2 \Big/ 3$$

$$= (2*(0.025 - 0.0333)^2 + (0.05 - 0.0333)^2) \Big/ 3 = 0.000139$$

$$\widehat{Var}(p_y) = (\widehat{SE}(p_y))^2 = (0.02849)^2 = 0.000812$$

The true variance of the sampling distribution, 0.000139, is smaller than the estimated variance, 0.000812, computed using the methods in part (b).

d.   *Suppose that a simple random sample of 40 homes had been selected instead. What is the variance of the distribution of the estimated proportion of lead hazardous homes in this case? How does this value compare with the variance from a 1 in 3 systematic sample?*

Solution: Assuming a simple random sample, $E(p_y) = P_y = 4/120 = 0.0333$

$$Var(p_y) = \frac{P_y(1 - P_y)}{n}\frac{N - n}{N - 1} = 0.00054 > 0.000139$$

The estimate of the variance under the simple random sampling design is larger than the one obtained under the systematic random sampling design.

4.2   *From the 120 homes of Exercise 1, suppose a 1 in 5 systematic sample was taken and suppose that the initial random number was 5.*

a.   *Estimate the proportion of homes with lead hazards from the sample.*

Solution: $N = 120$, $k = 5$, houses 26, 27, 28, 29 are affected, $n = N/k = 120/5 = 24$

If we start with house 5, we sample homes 5, 10, 15, 20, 25, 30, …

Our estimate of the proportion of homes with lead hazards is:

$$p_y = \frac{0}{24} = 0$$

b.   *Obtain a 95% confidence interval for the proportion of homes with lead hazards.*

Solution: Cannot compute an estimated 95% confidence interval because the estimated proportion is zero. Therefore, the estimate of the SE will be zero.

c.   *What is the true variance of the distribution of the estimated proportion of homes with lead hazards? How does this compare with the estimated variance you used in part (b)?*

Solution: The five possible values of p_y are $1/24 = 0.04167$, $1/24 = 0.04167$, $1/24 = 0.04167$, $1/24 = 0.04167$, and $0/24 = 0$.

$$E(p_y) = \left(\frac{1}{5}\right) * (0.04167 + 0.04167 + 0.04167 + 0.04167 + 0_- = 0.0333$$

$$Var(p_y) = \sum_{1}^{5} (p_y - E(p_y))^2 \Big/ 5$$

$$= ((4 * (0.04167 - 0.0333)^2 + (0 - 0.0333)^2) \Big/ 5 = 0.000278$$

$$\widehat{Var}(p_y) = (\widehat{SE}(p_y))^{1/2} = (0)^{1/2} = 0$$

The true variance of the sampling distribution, 0.000278, cannot be compared to that computed in part (b), since by chance we estimated a proportion of zero.

d.   *Suppose that instead of a 1 in 5 systematic sample, a simple random sample of the same number of homes is taken. What is the variance of the distribution of the estimated proportion of lead hazardous homes obtained from this sampling scheme? How does this value compare to that obtained from a 1 in 5 systematic sample?*

Solution: Assuming a simple random sample,

$$E(p_y) = \frac{4}{120} = 0.0333$$

$$Var(p_y) = \left(\frac{p_y(1 - p_y)}{n}\right) * \frac{N - n}{N - 1} = 0.00108$$

The estimate of the variance under a simple random sampling design, 0.00108, is larger than the one obtained under the systematic random sampling design, 0.000278.

4.3   *Refer again to Exercise 4.2. Suppose that instead of a 1 in 5 systematic sample, a total of 24 homes are obtained by repeated systematic sampling of 1 in 40 homes.*

a.   *Suppose that the random numbers chosen are 3, 7, 12, 26, 31, 33, 38, and 40. Estimate the proportion of homes with lead hazards and obtain a confidence interval for the estimated proportion.*

Solution:

Random Start	Sample Points	P_y
3	3,43,83	0.0000
7	7,47,87	0.0000
12	12,52,92	0.0000
26	26,66,106	0.3333
31	31,71,111	0.0000
33	33,73,113	0.0000
38	38,78,118	0.0000
40	40,80,120	0.0000

$M = 40$, $m = 8$, $p_y = 0.3333/8 = 0.04167$

The estimated 95% confidence interval can be computed using the formula in Box 4.3.

$$0.04167 \pm 1.96 * (0.04167 * 0.95833/7)^{1/2} * ((40 - 8)/40)^{1/2}$$
$$= 0.04167 \pm 1.96 * 0.037269 = 0.04167 \pm 0.07305$$

Our estimated 95% confidence interval is (0, 0.1147).

Using STATA:

```
. gen M = 40
. gen wt = M / 8

. list, clean

      propor~n   wt    M
  1.         0    5   40
  2.         0    5   40
  3.         0    5   40
  4.     .3333    5   40
  5.         0    5   40
  6.         0    5   40
  7.         0    5   40
  8.         0    5   40

. svyset _n [pweight=wt]

      pweight: wt
          VCE: linearized
  Single unit: missing
     Strata 1: <one>
         SU 1: <observations>
        FPC 1: <zero>

. svy: mean proportion
(running mean on estimation sample)

Survey: Mean estimation

Number of strata =        1        Number of obs    =        8
Number of PSUs   =        8        Population size  =       40
                                   Design df        =        7

-----------------------------------------------------------------
             |              Linearized
             |      Mean    Std. Err.     [95% Conf. Interval]
-------------+---------------------------------------------------
  proportion |  .0416625    .0416625     -.0568537    .1401787
-----------------------------------------------------------------
```

Note STATA confidence intervals differ from those obtained by Box 4.3 formulas because STATA in this instance does not recognize that lower limit cannot be below 0, and also STATA uses t-distribution to obtain confidence intervals rather than normal distribution.

b. *What is the estimated variance of the distribution of the estimated proportion of lead hazardous homes obtained from these eight systematic samples of 1 in 40 households? Compare this to the actual variance that arises from a 1 in 5 systematic sample, which you calculated in part(c) of Exercise 4.2.*

Solution: Estimated variance = $(0.0372678)^2 = 0.001389$

The true variance of the sampling distribution, 0.000278, was computed in Exercise 4.2, part(c). The true variance is much smaller than the estimated variance obtained using these eight systematic samples of 1 in 40.

4.4 *From the list of 162 workers in Table 4.17, use repeated systematic sampling to take a total sample of 18 workers for purpose of estimating the total number of work days lost due to acute illnesses by all workers and the proportion of workers having eight or more work days lost due to acute illness. Obtain 95% confidence intervals for each of these estimates. (Suppose that the random numbers you chose were 4, 44, 29, 20, 27, and 5.)*

Solution: We will take 6 systematic samples of 1 in 54 workers.

Random Start	Sample Points	x	p_y
4	4, 58, 112	26	0.667
44	44, 98, 152	16	0
29	29, 83, 137	8	0
20	20, 74, 128	20	0.333
27	27, 81, 135	18	0.333
5	5, 59, 113	17	0.333

Using STATA:

```
. gen M = 54
. gen wt1 = M/6

. svyset _n [pweight=wt1], fpc(M)

      pweight: wt1
          VCE: linearized
  Single unit: missing
     Strata 1: <one>
         SU 1: <observations>
        FPC 1: m
. list

      Cluster       x_i       p_y          M        wt1
   1.       4        26      .667         54          9
   2.      44        16         0         54          9
   3.      29         8         0         54          9
   4.      20        20      .333         54          9
   5.      27        18      .333         54          9
   6.       5        17      .333         54          9

. svy: total x_i
(running total on estimation sample)

Survey: Total estimation

Number of strata =        1      Number of obs   =        6
Number of PSUs   =        6      Population size =       54
                                 Design df       =        5

--------------------------------------------------------------
```

```
                    |              Linearized
                    |     Total    Std. Err.     [95% Conf. Interval]
--------------------+---------------------------------------------------
            x_i |      945    121.7276      632.0893    1257.911
--------------------------------------------------------------------------

. svyset _n [pweight=wt1], fpc(m)

      pweight: wt1
          VCE: linearized
  Single unit: missing
     Strata 1: <one>
        SU 1: <observations>
       FPC 1: m

. svy: total x_i
(running total on estimation sample)

Survey: Total estimation

Number of strata =          1       Number of obs    =         6
Number of PSUs   =          6       Population size  =        54
                                    Design df        =         5


                    |              Linearized
                    |     Total    Std. Err.     [95% Conf. Interval]
--------------------+---------------------------------------------------
            x_i |      945    121.7276      632.0893    1257.911
--------------------------------------------------------------------------

. svy: mean p_y
(running mean on estimation sample)

Survey: Mean estimation

Number of strata =          1       Number of obs    =         6
Number of PSUs   =          6       Population size  =        54
                                    Design df        =         5


                    |              Linearized
                    |      Mean    Std. Err.     [95% Conf. Interval]
--------------------+---------------------------------------------------
            p_y |  .2776667    .0966036      .0293393    .525994
--------------------------------------------------------------------------
```

Our estimate of the total number of work days lost due to acute illnesses by all workers is 945 and a 95% confidence interval for this estimate is (632,1258). The estimated proportion of all workers having eight or more work days lost due to acute illnesses is 0.28 and a 95% confidence interval for this estimate is (0.03, 0.53).

4.5   *Suppose that a study is planned of the level of the pesticide dieldrin, which is believed to be a carcinogen, in a 7.5 mile stretch of a particular river. To assure representativeness, a map of the river is divided into 36 zones (see map on page 115 in book), and a 1 in 4 systematic sample of these zones is to be selected. Water samples will be drawn by taking a boat out to the geographic center of the designated zone, and drawing a grab sample of water from a depth of several centimeters below the surface level. The levels of dieldrin, in micrograms per liter, for each of these zones are shown in parentheses.*

a.   *Compute the 90% confidence interval for the average level of dieldrin in this stretch of the river.*

Solution: Suppose our random start is chosen to be zone 2. Then, our sample will include zones 4, 8, 12, 16, 20, 24, 28, 32, 36.

Using STATA:

```
. list

        Zone   Dieldrin         N        wt
 1.        4          1        36         4
 2.        8          1        36         4
 3.       12          6        36         4
 4.       16          5        36         4
 5.       20          3        36         4
 6.       24          2        36         4
 7.       28          2        36         4
 8.       32          1        36         4
 9.       36          0        36         4

. gen N = 36

. gen wt = N / 9

. svyset _n [pweight=wt], fpc(N)

      pweight: wt
          VCE: linearized
 Single unit: missing
     Strata 1: <one>
        SU 1: <observations>
       FPC 1: N

. svy: mean  Dieldrin, level(90)
(running mean on estimation sample)

Survey: Mean estimation

Number of strata =        1        Number of obs    =        9
Number of PSUs   =        9        Population size  =       36
                                   Design df        =        8

-------------------------------------------------------------
             |            Linearized
             |     Mean   Std. Err.     [90% Conf. Interval]
-------------+-----------------------------------------------
    Dieldrin |  2.333333   .5773503      1.259723    3.406944
-------------------------------------------------------------
```

The estimated mean level of dieldrin in the river is 2.33 micrograms per liter and the estimated 90% confidence interval for the estimate is (1.26, 3.41).

b.   *What advantages can you identify for this method of sampling the river over simple random sampling?*

> **Solution:** The advantage of using systematic random sampling is that we are assured that all stretches of the river are sampled. With simple random sampling, it is possible that only sections upstream, midstream or downstream would be sampled. If levels are thought to vary over the length of the river, then systematic random sampling is the method to use.

4.6   *During a specific year, 200 cardiac catheterization procedures were performed on persons over 70 years of age at a large university hospital. From a list of these patients, 4 systematic samples of 1 in 50 patients yielded the following data relating to pulmonary artery pressure.*

Sample	Individual	Mean Pulmonary Artery Pressure
1	30	16
	80	25
	130	15
	180	17
2	17	14
	67	19
	117	18
	167	20
3	22	19
	72	27
	122	30
	172	11
4	43	10
	93	33
	143	17
	193	13

Based on these preliminary data, how many repeated systematic samples of 1 in 50 persons would have to be taken in order to estimate the mean pulmonary pressure in this population to within 10% of the true mean?

Solution: $M' = 50$, $m' = 4$, $\varepsilon = 0.1$ $N/n = 200/4 = 50$

Using $z = 1.96$ (95% certainty), we have from equation (4.11):

$$m = \frac{1.96^2 * \frac{3.41667}{19^2} * 50}{(50 - 1) * (0.1)^2 + 1.96^2 * \frac{3.41667}{19^2}} = 3.45 \approx 4$$

4.7   *The following represents a week of scheduled appointments for the staff dentist at a small community health center characterized by major activity (B = Basic Care; C = Comprehensive Care):*

Week 1	Mon	Tue	Wed	Thur	Fri
9:00	B	B	B	B	B
10:00	B	C	C	C	B
11:00	B	C	B	C	B
1:00	C	C	C	B	C
2:00	C	C	B	C	B
3:00	B	B	B	B	B
4:00	B	B	B	B	B

It is desired to estimate the proportion of visits devoted to comprehensive care during a particular 52-week period by use of a sampling plan involving systematic sampling. A 1 in 7 systematic sample is proposed. Is this a good sampling plan in this situation? Why or why not?

Solution: No, this is not a good sampling plan. In the sample week, the first appointment (9:00 am) and the last two (3:00 pm and 4:00 pm) are all basic care. If a 1 in 7 systematic scheme were used, this would result in periodicities and an estimate having large standard error.

4.8   *During a 52-week period there are 1820 (35*52) appointment slots in the situation described in Exercise 4.7. A repeated systematic sampling design of 1 in 26 appointment slots is to be used to estimate the proportion of appointments devoted to comprehensive care during that 52-week period. A pilot study of 3 such 1 in 26 samples yielded the following results:*

Sample	Proportion Comprehensive
1	12/70
2	23/70
3	18/70

Based on the above results, how many replicated 1 in 26 samples would be required in order to be 95% certain of estimating this proportion to within 10% of the true value.

Solution: $m' = 3$, $\varepsilon = 0.1$, $N/n = 1820/70 = 26$

Using $z = 1.96$ (95% certainty), we have from equation (4.11):

$$m = \frac{1.96^2 * \dfrac{0.006191}{190.2524^2} * 26}{(26-1) * (0.1)^2 + 1.96^2 * \dfrac{0.006191}{0.2524^2}} = 15.57 \approx 16$$

4.9   *Which of the following is not true about systematic sampling?*

   a. Variances of estimates are large when the sampling ratio coincides with a periodicity in the frame.

   b. Variances of estimates are related to the size of the intraclass correlation coefficient.

   c. Unlike simple random sampling, one does not need to know the number of elements in the population in order to perform systematic sampling.

   d. Estimated means, totals, and proportions are always unbiased under systematic sampling.

   Solution: Statement *d* is not true. Unbiased estimates result when *k* is an integer.

4.10   *Systematic sampling works best under which of the following scenarios?*

   a. The sampling frame (or list) is ordered with respect to a variable that is directly related to and highly correlated with the variable of interest.

   b. The sampling frame is neither ordered nor has any periodicity with respect to any variable of interest.

   c. The sampling frame has a periodicity in it that is congruent with the sampling fraction.

   d. The sampling frame is not a list.

   Solution: Scenario *a* is the best one because this results in an estimate with a small variance.

4.11   *Suppose that in the scenario of Exercise 4.1, it is decided to take a sample of 18 homes according to a repeated systematic sampling design which specifies 6 replications of a systematic sample of 3 homes.*

a.   *In the notation developed in this chapter for repeated systematic sampling, specify N, M, n and m. What is the numerical value of the sampling weight?*

Solution: $N = 120$, $M = 40$, $n = 3$, $m = 6$
The numerical value of the sampling weight is 40/6 or 6.667.

b.   *Suppose that the 6 random numbers chosen for the sampling design specified in part a are: 3, 15, 20, 27, 34, and 39. Which households appear in the sample?*

Solution:

Random Start	Households	P_y
3	3,43,83	0.0000
15	15,45,85	0.0000
20	20,60,100	0.0000
27	27,67,107	0.3333
34	34,74,114	0.0000
39	39,79,119	0.0000

c.   *(For those having access to SUDAAN or STATA) From the sample taken in part b, use SUDAAN or STATA to estimate the number and proportion of homes having lead hazards and the standard errors of these estimates.*

Solution:

```
. gen M = 40
. gen wt1 = M/6
. list
     Cluster    Proportion      x_i        M        wt1
  1.        3            0        0        40    6.666667
  2.       15            0        0        40    6.666667
  3.       20            0        0        40    6.666667
  4.       27        .3333        1        40    6.666667
  5.       34            0        0        40    6.666667
  6.       39            0        0        40    6.666667

. svyset _n [pweight=wt1], fpc(M)

      pweight: wt1
          VCE: linearized
  Single unit: missing
     Strata 1: <one>
         SU 1: <observations>
```

```
          FPC 1: M
. svy: total x_i
(running total on estimation sample)

Survey: Total estimation

Number of strata =          1        Number of obs    =        6
Number of PSUs   =          6        Population size  =       40
                                     Design df        =        5

-----------------------------------------------------------------
             |              Linearized
             |    Total     Std. Err.     [95% Conf. Interval]
-------------+---------------------------------------------------
       x_i |  6.666667     6.146363      -9.133063    22.4664
-----------------------------------------------------------------
. svy: mean  Proportion
(running mean on estimation sample)

Survey: Mean estimation

Number of strata =          1        Number of obs    =        6
Number of PSUs   =          6        Population size  =       40
                                     Design df        =        5
-----------------------------------------------------------------
             |              Linearized
             |    Mean      Std. Err.     [95% Conf. Interval]
-------------+---------------------------------------------------
 proportion |   .05555      .0512146     -.0761012    .1872012
-----------------------------------------------------------------
```

The estimated total number of homes having lead hazards is 6.67 and the standard error of this estimate is 6.15. The estimated proportion of homes having lead hazards is 0.056 and the standard error of this estimate is 0.051.

4.12 *A data file contains 100,000 records on 2012 members of a health maintenance organization (HMO). Records are labeled beginning with "1" and ending with "100,000" and a random number is selected between 1 and 1000. The random number selected is 253, and all records ending with 253 are sampled (e.g. 253, 1253, 2253, 3253, etc.). For each record selected, the HMO member corresponding to each sample record is queried concerning his/her risk factors for coronary heart disease. An estimate of the proportion of persons at high risk for coronary heart disease (CHD) is then constructed by use of the sample proportion (number of persons at high risk divided by number of persons in the sample).*

a. *The sample proportion described above is a biased estimate of the true population proportion. Show why this is true.*

Solution: Records are the enumeration unit, whereas HMO members are the units of analysis. If the number of records is not the same for each individual, then the chances of an individual being in the sample is proportional to the number of records in the individual's file. An ordinary proportion does not take this into consideration and hence is not an unbiased estimate.

b. *Construct an unbiased estimate for this sample design.*

Solution: Weight each individual's value by the reciprocal of the person's number of records in the file in order to get an unbiased estimate.

4.13   The sample described in Exercise 4.12 yields the following data on the 100 HMO enrollees selected as described above. From these data estimate the proportion of persons in the HMO population at high risk for coronary heart disease.

Solution: We list the first 20 individuals sampled.

```
. list in 1/20

        rec_num     num_rec    chdhirsk
 1.        253          50          0
 2.       1253          36          0
 3.       2253          45          0
 4.       3253          61          0
 5.       4253          50          0
 6.       5253          77          0
 7.       6253          70          0
 8.       7253          41          0
 9.       8253          63          0
10.       9253          43          0
11.      10253          53          0
12.      11253          17          1
13.      12253          44          0
14.      13253          54          0
15.      14253          70          0
16.      15253          46          0
17.      16253          62          0
18.      17253          48          0
19.      18253          37          0
20.      19253          53          0
```

The chance of an individual being selected is proportional to the number of records for the individual that are in the file of 100,000 records. Since there are 100 records in the sample, the probability of an individual being selected in the sample is approximately equal to (*num_rec*/100,000)*100 where *num_rec* is the number of records for the individual in the file of 100,00 records (see pages 494-495 of text for demonstration of this). The appropriate sample weight would then be the reciprocal of this expression. We generate this weight, called *wt*.

```
. gen wt = 100000 / (num_rec*100)

. sum chdhirsk [w=wt]
(analytic weights assumed)

    Variable |     Obs      Weight        Mean   Std. Dev.        Min        Max
-------------+--------------------------------------------------------------------
    chdhirsk |     100   2505.61313    .2878506    .455042          0          1
```

The unbiased estimate of the proportion having CHD risk is 0.2879, which is more than double the unweighted mean, 0.14.

Chapter Five – Solutions

5.1   *From a simple random serological sample of 1000 runners selected from 10,000 who completed the 1995 Chicago Marathon, 35 were found to be positive for steroids and other performance-enhancing drugs. When categorized by completion time, the results were as follows:*

Completion Time (h)	No. in Sample	No. Positive for Drugs	Percentage Positive
Under 2.5	100	25	25.00
2.5-4.0	500	7	1.40
Over 4.0	400	3	0.75
Total	1000	35	3.50

a.   *What is the standard error of the estimated proportion positive?*

Solution: Assuming simple random sampling, the standard error of the estimate is equal to

$$\widehat{SE}(p_y) = \sqrt{\frac{N-n}{N}}\sqrt{\frac{p_y(1-p_y)}{n-1}} = \sqrt{\frac{9000}{10000}}\sqrt{\frac{0.033775}{999}} = 0.005516$$

b.   *From inspection (without making calculations) of the rates given above, would you feel that stratification may have resulted in a substantially better estimate? Why or why not?*

Solution: Stratification would have likely resulted in a better estimate because the proportion of runners who tested positive is much higher in the "Under 2.5" group compared to the other two groups. Thus, stratifying on time will produce homogeneous within-strata and heterogeneous between-strata estimates, leading to an estimate with a lower standard error than that obtained from simple random sampling. Also, stratified sampling will assure that there are enough people in the "Under 2.5" group to obtain a stable estimate.

5.2　*Suppose that in the situation of Exercise 5.1, of the 10,000 completing the marathon, 2000 completed the event in less than 2.5 h; 6000 completed the event in 2.5-4.0 h; and 2000 completed the event in more than 4 h. Comment on the results of the sampling as given in Exercise 5.1.*

Solution: In the population, 20% of the runners completed the event in less than 2.5 hours, whereas in our sample, only 10% of such runners were included. Also, in the true population, 60% of the runners finished between 2.5 and 4 hours and 20% completed the marathon in more than 4 hours, however the sample contained 50% and 40%, respectively, of these runners. A much larger proportion of the runners who ran in under 2.5 hours tested positive, compared to the other groups, and they were underrepresented in the sample. Furthermore, the runners who had times that were greater than 4 hours had a lower proportion of positive tests, compared to the other groups, and they were overrepresented in the sample. The resulting estimate is likely an underestimate of the truth owing to the fact that the proportions of fast, intermediate and slower runners did not reflect the population proportions and the likelihood of testing positive appears to vary with finish time.

5.3　*If a stratified random sample of 333 persons in each of the three groups had been taken, what would likely be the resulting estimated percentage positive?*

Solution: If we conducted a stratified sample, and assumed that the same proportions of positive tests are found in the stratified design, then we can use the equation in Box 5.2 to estimate the proportion positive in the entire population:

$$p_{y,str} = \frac{\sum_{h=1}^{L} y_{hi}}{N} = \frac{2000 * 0.25 + 6000 * 0.014 + 2000 * 0.0075}{10{,}000} = 0.0599 \; or \; 5.99\,\%$$

5.4   *An additional 2000 runners entered the race but did not complete it. Of these runners, a mail questionnaire was sent to a random sample of 600 and completed by 500. One of the items in this questionnaire asked the respondent to estimate the average number of miles run weekly during the 8 weeks preceding the marathon. The mean of the number of miles run was 32.4 with standard deviation equal to 7.3. A simple random sample of 500 of the 10,000 runners completing the marathon yielded 400 respondents who averaged 46.8 miles weekly with standard deviation equal to 6.2 miles. What is the average weekly miles run in that period among all those who entered the marathon?*

Solution: Using the formula in Box 5.2 for estimating a mean from a stratified random sample,

$$\bar{x}_{str} = \frac{\sum_{h=1}^{L} N_h \bar{x}_h}{N} = \frac{2000 * 32.4 + 10,000 * 46.8}{12,000} = 44.4 \ miles \ per \ week$$

5.5   *The following data are available for 2007 for 6 Health Maintenance Organizations (HMOs) in a medium-size city:*

Number of personnel providing patient care and number of patient encounters during 1988 among six HMOs

HMO	No. of Physicians Providing Patient Care	No. of Patient Encounters
1	10	22,000
2	6	14,000
3	4	10,200
4	30	70,000
5	7	15,000
6	3	5,000

As a time- and cost-sharing device, it is proposed that a sample of two of these HMOs be taken for purposes of estimating the total number of patient encounters in 2008 among these six HMOs.

a.   *Enumerate all simple random samples of size 2 and estimate the total number of patient encounters in 2008 among the 6 HMOs.*

Solution: The 15 samples are included in the following table.

Sample	Total in sample HMO 1	Total in sample HMO 2	Estimated Population Total
1, 2	22,000	14,000	108,000
1, 3	22,000	10,200	96,600
1, 4	22,000	70,000	276,000
1, 5	22,000	15,000	111,000
1, 6	22,000	5,000	81,000
2, 3	14,000	10,200	72,600
2, 4	14,000	70,000	252,000
2, 5	14,000	15,000	87,000
2, 6	14,000	5,000	57,000
3, 4	10,200	70,000	240,600
3, 5	10,200	15,000	75,600
3, 6	10,200	5,000	45,600
4, 5	70,000	15,000	255,000
4, 6	70,000	5,000	225,000
5, 6	15,000	5,000	60,000

b.   *What is the standard error of the estimated total from the sample design specified above?*

Solution: Using STATA, the standard deviation of the total from the 15 samples is 82592.5 patient encounters.

```
. sum total

    Variable |      Obs       Mean    Std. Dev.       Min        Max
-------------+--------------------------------------------------------
       total |       15     136200    85491.35      45600     276000

. display (85491.35*sqrt(14/15))
82592.491
```

c.   *Group HMOs 1, 2, 3, 5, and 6 into 1 stratum and HMO 4 into another (by itself). From these two strata, enumerate all stratified random samples of size 2. What is the standard error of the estimated total as obtained by this sampling plan?*

Solution: The five samples are included in the following table.

Sample	Total in sample HMO 1	Total in sample HMO 2	Estimated Population Total
1, 4	22,000	70,000	180,000
2, 4	14,000	70,000	140,000
3, 4	10,200	70,000	121,000
5, 4	15,000	70,000	145,000
6, 4	5,000	70,000	95,000

```
. sum total

    Variable |      Obs       Mean   Std. Dev.       Min        Max
-------------+--------------------------------------------------------
       total |        5     136200   31379.93      95000     180000

. display (31379.93*sqrt(4/5))
28067.063
```

The standard deviation of the total of this sampling distribution is 28067.1 patient encounters.

d.   *Comment on the utility of using stratification in this situation as opposed to simple random sampling.*

Solution: Clearly, the stratified sampling scheme results in an estimate with greater precision. The standard deviation of the sampling distribution is 28067.1, which is much smaller than the standard deviation using simple random sampling, 82592.5 patient encounters. This is due to the fact that there are fewer visits among HMOs in stratum 1 compared to the HMO in stratum 2.

5.6   *Suppose that in the situation given in Exercise 5.5 it is desired to estimate the number of encounters per physician in 2008. Repeat parts (a)-(d) in Exercise 5.5 for this situation. Is stratified random sampling superior to simple random sampling in this situation? Why is it or why is it not?*

a.   *Enumerate all simple random samples of size 2 and estimate the number of encounters per physician in 2008 among the 6 HMOs.*

Solution: The 15 samples are included in the following table.

Sample	Total in sample HMO 1	Total in sample HMO 2	Estimated Population Total
1, 2	10	6	48
1, 3	10	4	42
1, 4	10	30	120
1, 5	10	7	51
1, 6	10	3	39
2, 3	6	4	30
2, 4	6	30	108
2, 5	6	7	39
2, 6	6	3	27
3, 4	4	30	102
3, 5	4	7	33
3, 6	4	3	21
4, 5	30	7	111
4, 6	30	3	99
5, 6	7	3	20

b.   *What is the standard error of the estimated total from the sample design specified above?*

> **Solution:** Using STATA, the standard deviation of the total from the 15 samples is 109.3 patient encounters per physician.

```
. list

             S1        S2       totmd       totvisit
  1.         10         6          48         108000
  2.         10         4          42          96600
  3.         10        30         120         276000
  4.         10         7          51         111000
  5.         10         3          39          81000
  6.          6         4          30          72600
  7.          6        30         108         252000
  8.          6         7          39          87000
  9.          6         3          27          57000
 10.          4        30         102         240600
 11.          4         7          33          75600
 12.          4         3          21          45600
 13.         30         7         111         255000
 14.         30         3          99         225000
 15.          7         3          30          60000

. gen enctphys = totvisit / totmd

. sum enctphys

    Variable |     Obs        Mean    Std. Dev.        Min        Max
-------------+------------------------------------------------------
    enctphys |      15     2239.32    113.1051       2000       2420


. display (113.1051*sqrt(14/15))
109.26991
```

c.   *Group HMOs 1, 2, 3, 5, and 6 into 1 stratum and HMO 4 into another (by itself). From these two strata, enumerate all stratified random samples of size 2. What is the standard error of the estimated total per physician as obtained by this sampling plan?*

> **Solution:** The five samples are included in the following table.

Sample	Total in sample HMO 1	Total in sample HMO 2	Estimated Population Total
1, 4	10	30	80
2, 4	6	30	60
3, 4	4	30	50
5, 4	7	30	65
6, 4	3	30	45

```
. list

            S1        S2      totmd      totvisit
 1.         10        30        80        180000
 2.          6        30        60        140000
 3.          4        30        50        121000
 4.          7        30        65        145000
 5.          3        30        45         95000

. gen enctphys = totvisit / totmd

. sum enctphys

    Variable |     Obs        Mean   Std. Dev.         Min         Max
-------------+--------------------------------------------------------
    enctphys |       5    2269.043   115.8569    2111.111        2420

. display (115.8561*sqrt(4/5))
103.62485
```

The standard deviation of the total of this sampling distribution is 103.6 patient encounters per physician.

d.   *Comment on the utility of using stratification in this situation as opposed to simple random sampling.*

Solution: The standard deviation of the distribution of the estimated total encounters per physician from stratified random sampling, 103.6, does not differ much from that obtained from simple random sampling, 109.3. The reason is because there is not much variability in the number of encounters per physician among the six HMOs. This demonstrates that while stratified sampling may be more efficient in some settings, it is not the best method for sampling in all situations.

5.7   *In a large clinic located in an inner city hospital, 56 patients with nonsymptomatic HIV infection have been treated with an experimental drug believed to have the capability of restoring certain immune system functions associated with HIV infection. Of these patients, 12 had CD4 cell counts below 250 at the initial visit; 20 had counts between 250 and 400; and 24 had counts above 400. (The lower the count, the worse the prognosis.) It is desired to take a stratified random sample of the 30 patients, 10 from each of the three groups described above, for purposes of estimating the 12-month incidence of AIDS-defining events among these patients.*

a.   *How many samples of 30 patients taken as described above are possible?*

Solution: $\binom{12}{10} \times \binom{20}{10} \times \binom{24}{10} = 2.391535169 \times 10^{13}$

b.   *Assuming that a patient can have more than one AIDS-defining event during this period, show algebraically how you would estimate the 12-month incidence of AIDS-defining events from the sample.*

Solution: The incidence is defined as the number of events divided by the total number of persons. Algebraically, this is equivalent to finding a population total for the 12-month period, and then expressing that total as a total per 56 persons. We can estimate the mean number of events in each stratum, and then inflate the means according to the number of patients per stratum. Then, we can sum the estimated totals and express them as the total number of events per 56 persons.

$$\text{Incidence} = 12x_1 + 20x_2 + 24x_3 / 56,$$

where x_1, x_2, and x_3 are the number of events in stratum 1, stratum 2, and stratum 3, respectively.

c.   *How many samples of size 30 are possible under simple random sampling without stratification?*

Solution: (56 choose 30) $= 6.646448384 \times 10^{15}$

5.8   *The results of the sample survey described in Exercise 5.7 are shown below:*

	Number of Persons		
Number of Events	*CD4 < 250*	*250 ≤ CD4 < 400*	*CD4 ≥ 400*
0	*5*	*7*	*9*
1	*1*	*2*	*1*
2	*2*	*1*	*0*
3	*2*	*0*	*0*

From these data, estimate the incidence of AIDS defining events in the target population. What is the standard error of the estimated incidence rate? (You have to derive the formula for the standard error from "first principles.")

Solution: We need to create a STATA data set containing data on the group and number of events for each patient in the sample.

```
. gen N = 12

. replace N = 20 if Group == 2
(10 real changes made)

. replace N = 24 if Group == 3
(10 real changes made)

. gen wt1 = N / 10

. svyset _n [pweight=wt], fpc(N) strata(Group)

      pweight: wt1
          VCE: linearized
  Single unit: missing
     Strata 1: Group
         SU 1: <observations>
        FPC 1: N

. list

        Group    Events        N      wt1
  1.        1         0       12      1.2
  2.        1         0       12      1.2
  3.        1         0       12      1.2
  4.        1         0       12      1.2
  5.        1         0       12      1.2
  6.        1         1       12      1.2
  7.        1         2       12      1.2
  8.        1         2       12      1.2
  9.        1         3       12      1.2
 10.        1         3       12      1.2
 11.        2         0       20        2
 12.        2         0       20        2
 13.        2         0       20        2
```

14.	2	0	20	2
15.	2	0	20	2
16.	2	0	20	2
17.	2	0	20	2
18.	2	1	20	2
19.	2	1	20	2
20.	2	2	20	2
21.	3	0	24	2.4
22.	3	0	24	2.4
23.	3	0	24	2.4
24.	3	0	24	2.4
25.	3	0	24	2.4
26.	3	0	24	2.4
27.	3	0	24	2.4
28.	3	0	24	2.4
29.	3	0	24	2.4
30.	3	1	24	2.4

```
. svy: mean Events
(running mean on estimation sample)

Survey: Mean estimation

Number of strata =          3      Number of obs    =        30
Number of PSUs   =         30      Population size  =        56
                                   Design df        =        27

--------------------------------------------------------------
             |             Linearized
             |      Mean   Std. Err.     [95% Conf. Interval]
-------------+------------------------------------------------
      Events |  .4214286   .0738671      .2698658    .5729914
--------------------------------------------------------------
```

The estimated incidence rate is 0.42 events per person. The standard error of this estimate is 0.07

5.9 *From the data in Exercise 5.8, estimate the proportion of patients having one or more AIDS-defining events. What is the standard error of this estimated proportion?*

Solution: Using STATA, we can calculate this proportion. First, we must create a new variable called event_1 which will take on the value of 1 if the person has one or more event, and zero if no events are experienced.

```
. gen event_1=(Events>0)

. tab event_1

    event_1 |      Freq.      Percent        Cum.
------------+-----------------------------------
          0 |         21        70.00       70.00
          1 |          9        30.00      100.00
------------+-----------------------------------
      Total |         30       100.00

. svy: mean event_1
(running mean on estimation sample)

Survey: Mean estimation

Number of strata =        3        Number of obs     =       30
Number of PSUs   =       30        Population size   =       56
                                   Design df         =       27


-----------------------------------------------------------------
            |               Linearized
            |      Mean    Std. Err.      [95% Conf. Interval]
------------+----------------------------------------------------
    event_1 |  .2571429    .0526508       .1491123    .3651734
-----------------------------------------------------------------
```

The estimated proportion of patients who have one or more AIDS-defining event is 0.26 and the standard error of this estimate is 0.05.

5.10   *A simple random sample (without stratification) of 30 of these 56 patients yielded the following data:*

Number of Events	CD4 < 250	250 ≤ CD4 < 400	CD4 ≥ 400
		Number of Persons	
0	3	8	12
1	1	2	0
2	0	1	1
3	2	0	0

Estimate the incidence of AIDS-defining events from these data and the standard error of this estimate. Compare this to the results obtained from the stratified sampling design. Which design produces the more reliable estimate? Why does it?

Solution: Using STATA, we have to create a data set containing group membership and the number of events. Then we can estimate the incidence rate assuming simple random sampling.

```
. gen N = 56

. gen wt1 = N / 30

. list

          Group    Events        N       wt1
   1.        1        0          56    1.866667
   2.        1        0          56    1.866667
   3.        1        0          56    1.866667
   4.        1        1          56    1.866667
   5.        1        3          56    1.866667
   6.        1        3          56    1.866667
   7.        2        0          56    1.866667
   8.        2        0          56    1.866667
   9.        2        0          56    1.866667
  10.        2        0          56    1.866667
  11.        2        0          56    1.866667
  12.        2        0          56    1.866667
  13.        2        0          56    1.866667
  14.        2        0          56    1.866667
  15.        2        1          56    1.866667
  16.        2        1          56    1.866667
  17.        2        2          56    1.866667
  18.        3        0          56    1.866667
  19.        3        0          56    1.866667
  20.        3        0          56    1.866667
  21.        3        0          56    1.866667
  22.        3        0          56    1.866667
  23.        3        0          56    1.866667
  24.        3        0          56    1.866667
  25.        3        0          56    1.866667
  26.        3        0          56    1.866667
  27.        3        0          56    1.866667
  28.        3        0          56    1.866667
  29.        3        0          56    1.866667
  30.        3        2          56    1.866667
```

```
. svyset _n [pweight=wt1], fpc(N)

      pweight: wt1
          VCE: linearized
  Single unit: missing
     Strata 1: <one>
         SU 1: <observations>
        FPC 1: n

. svy: mean Events
(running mean on estimation sample)

Survey: Mean estimation

Number of strata =          1        Number of obs    =       30
Number of PSUs   =         30        Population size  =       56
                                     Design df        =       29

------------------------------------------------------------------
                 |               Linearized
                 |      Mean    Std. Err.     [95% Conf. Interval]
-----------------+------------------------------------------------
          Events |  .4333333    .1116687      .2049452    .6617214
------------------------------------------------------------------
```

Assuming a simple random sampling design, the estimated incidence rate is 0.43 and the standard error of this estimate is 0.11. In the stratified design, the estimated incidence rate was 0.42, with a standard error of 0.07. While the point estimates are similar, the standard error from stratified sampling is smaller than that obtained from simple random sampling. This occurs because the groups, defined by CD4 count, are different with respect to the number of AIDS-defining events experienced by patients.

Chapter Six – Solutions

6.1 *A sample survey of households in a community containing 1500 households is to be conducted for the purpose of determining the total number of persons over 18 years of age in the community who have one or more permanent teeth (other than third molars) missing. Since this variable is thought to be correlated with age and income, the strata shown in the accompanying table are formed by using available population data. A stratified random sample of 100 families is to be taken.*

		Stratum			
Variable		1	2	3	4
Age					
Mean		30	32	25	27
Standard deviation		15	15	10	10
Annual family income (x $1000)					
Mean		15	7	15	8
Standard deviation		5	3	3	2
No. of families		300	500	100	600

a. *Specify in algebraic detail how the estimate of the total number of persons having one or more missing teeth is to be estimated.*

Solution: We have to define an indicator variable, x_{hi}, which takes on the value of 1 if the sample person in stratum h has one or more missing teeth, and 0 if the person has no missing teeth.

$$\hat{x}_{str} = \sum_{h=1}^{L} \left(N_h / n_h\right) \sum_{i=1}^{n_h} x_{hi}$$

b. *Determine the number of families to be taken from each stratum if proportional allocation is used.*

Solution: In proportional allocation, the sampling fraction is the same for each stratum. Thus, the overall sampling fraction is the fraction taken from each stratum. From equation 6.9 on page 153 in the book:

$$n_h = N_h * (n / N)$$

In this problem, $n = 100$ and $N = 1500$.

$n_1 = 300 * (100 / 1500) = 20$
$n_2 = 500 * (100 / 1500) = 33.33$ or 33
$n_3 = 100 * (100 / 1500) = 6.67$ or 7
$n_4 = 600 * (100 / 1500) = 40$

c.   *Determine the number of families to be taken from each stratum if optimal allocation is used based on annual family income.*

Solution: Optimal allocation is used when the investigators believe that the variance obtained with proportional allocation can be improved upon. That is, optimal allocation will result in an estimate with lower variance than the estimate obtained with proportional allocation. From equation 6.17 on page 160 in the book:

$$n_h = \left(\frac{N_h \sigma_{hx}}{\sum_{h=1}^{L} N_h \sigma_{hx}} \right) (n)$$

$$n_1 = \frac{300 * 5}{(300 * 5) + (500 * 3) + (100 * 3) + (600 * 2)} * 100 = 33.33 \approx 33$$

$$n_2 = \frac{500 * 3}{(300 * 5) + (500 * 3) + (100 * 3) + (600 * 2)} * 100 = 33.33 \approx 33$$

$$n_3 = \frac{100 * 3}{(300 * 5) + (500 * 3) + (100 * 3) + (600 * 2)} * 100 = 6.67 \approx 7$$

$$n_4 = \frac{600 * 2}{(300 * 5) + (500 * 3) + (100 * 3) + (600 * 2)} * 100 = 26.67 \approx 27$$

d.   *Determine the number of families to be taken from each stratum if optimal allocation is used based on age.*

Solution: Optimal allocation is used when the investigators believe that the variance obtained with proportional allocation can be improved upon. That is, optimal allocation will result in an estimate with lower variance than the estimate obtained with proportional allocation.

$$n_1 = \frac{300 * 15}{(300 * 15) + (500 * 15) + (100 * 10) + (600 * 10)} * 100 = 23.68 \approx 24$$

$$n_2 = \frac{500 * 15}{(300 * 15) + (500 * 15) + (100 * 10) + (600 * 10)} * 100 = 39.47 \approx 39$$

$$n_3 = \frac{100 * 10}{(300 * 15) + (500 * 15) + (100 * 10) + (600 * 10)} * 100 = 5.26 \approx 5$$

$$n_4 = \frac{600 * 10}{(300 * 15) + (500 * 15) + (100 * 10) + (600 * 10)} * 100 = 31.57 \approx 32$$

e.   *How would you allocate sample to strata, taking into consideration both age and annual family income?*

Solution: One strategy would be to take the mean of the two sample sizes calculated from the two optimal allocation procedures.

$n_1 = (33 + 24) / 2 = 28.5 \approx 29$
$n_2 = (33 + 39) / 2 = 36$
$n_3 = (7 + 5) / 2 = 6$
$n_4 = (27 + 32) / 2 = 29.5 \approx 29$

f.   *What is the variance of the distribution of annual family income for the entire*
population?

> **Solution:** Using equations 6.13 and 6.15, the variance can be computed the following
> way:

$$\bar{x} = \frac{[(300 * 15) + (500 * 7) + (100 * 15) + (600 * 8)]}{1500} = 9.53$$

$$\sigma_{bx}^2 = \frac{(300(15 - 9.53)^2) + (500(7 - 9.53)^2) + (100(15 - 9.53)^2) + (600(8 - 9.53)^2)}{1500}$$
$$= 11.049$$

$$\sigma_{wx}^2 = \frac{[(300 * 5^2) + (500 * 3^2) + (100 * 3^2) + (600 * 2^2)]}{1500} = 10.2$$

$$\sigma_x^2 = \sigma_{wx}^2 + \sigma_{bx}^2 = 11.049 + 10.2$$

g.   *Suppose the number of persons over 18 years of age having missing teeth in a family is*
highly correlated with family income. Is stratified random sampling with proportional
allocation likely to yield an estimate having lower variance than that obtained from a
simple random sample of the same number of households?

> **Solution:** Yes, the variance obtained from stratified random sampling will be lower than
> that obtained from simple random sampling because the between-stratum variance, σ_{bx}^2,
> will always be less than σ_x^2.

6.2   *Let us suppose that the data from Table 3.8 were obtained from a stratified random*
sample of the 1200 workers in the plant in which the working force was stratified
according to pulmonary stressors (low, medium, high) and that proportional allocation
was used to allocate the sample.

a.   *How many workers are there in each stratum?*

> **Solution:** Using equation 6.9:

$n_1 = 6 = N_h(40/1200), N_1 = 180$
$n_2 = 6 = N_h(40/1200), N_2 = 180$
$n_3 = 28 = N_h(40/1200), N_3 = 840$

b.   *Estimate the mean forced vital capacity among the workers in the plant. How does this estimate differ from the mean that would have been obtained if the sample had been taken by simple random sampling?*

Solution: Using the sampling procedures for a stratified random in STATA:

```
. list

        worker    exposure         fvc      popsize          wt1
 1.         22           1          64         1200           30
 2.         21           2          70         1200           30
 3.         31           3          84         1200           30
 4.          7           1          82         1200           30
 5.         20           2          99         1200           30
 6.         33           3          89         1200           30
 7.          1           3          81         1200           30
 8.          8           1          99         1200           30
 9.         11           1          71         1200           30
10.         24           2          72         1200           30
11.         15           3          77         1200           30
12.         26           3          96         1200           30
13.         17           3          62         1200           30
14.         12           3          88         1200           30
15.         30           1          87         1200           30
16.         13           2          84         1200           30
17.         25           3          95         1200           30
18.         27           3          62         1200           30
19.         28           3          67         1200           30
20.         19           3          91         1200           30
21.         38           3          98         1200           30
22.          4           2          91         1200           30
23.          2           3          64         1200           30
24.         18           3          67         1200           30
25.         37           3          80         1200           30
26.          3           2          85         1200           30
27.         34           3          65         1200           30
28.          5           3          60         1200           30
29.         29           3          95         1200           30
30.         35           3          67         1200           30
31.         36           3          69         1200           30
32.         39           3          65         1200           30
33.         16           3          76         1200           30
34.          9           3          96         1200           30
35.         10           3          91         1200           30
36.          6           1          97         1200           30
37.         14           3          85         1200           30
38.         40           3          84         1200           30
39.         32           3          89         1200           30
40.         23           3          72         1200           30
```

Stratified Random Sampling

```
. gen N=840
. replace N=180 if exposure < 3
(12 real changes made)
. gen wt = N/6
. replace wt = N/28 if exposure == 3
(28 real changes made)

. svyset _n [pweight=wt], fpc(N) strata(exposure)

      pweight: wt
          VCE: linearized
  Single unit: missing
     Strata 1: exposure
        SU 1: <observations>
       FPC 1: N

. svy: mean fvc
(running mean on estimation sample)

Survey: Mean estimation

Number of strata =          3      Number of obs     =        40
Number of PSUs   =         40      Population size   =      1200
                                   Design df         =        37


-----------------------------------------------------------------
             |               Linearized
             |      Mean     Std. Err.     [95% Conf. Interval]
-------------+---------------------------------------------------
         fvc |      80.4     1.95447      76.43987      84.36013
-----------------------------------------------------------------
```

Simple Random Sampling

```
. gen N = 1200
. gen wt1 = N/40
. svyset _n [pweight=wt1], fpc(N)

      pweight: wt1
          VCE: linearized
  Single unit: missing
     Strata 1: <one>
        SU 1: <observations>
       FPC 1: N

. svy: mean fvc
(running mean on estimation sample)

Survey: Mean estimation

Number of strata =          1      Number of obs     =        40
Number of PSUs   =         40      Population size   =      1200
                                   Design df         =        39


-----------------------------------------------------------------
             |               Linearized
             |      Mean     Std. Err.     [95% Conf. Interval]
-------------+---------------------------------------------------
         fvc |      80.4     1.928777     76.49868      84.30132
-----------------------------------------------------------------
```

The estimated mean forced vital capacity among the workers in the plant is 80.4, which is the same as the mean that would have been obtained from a simple random sampling design because proportional allocation is self-weighting.

c.   *Obtain a 95% confidence interval for the population mean.*

Solution: From the STATA output, the 95% confidence interval for the forced vital capacity is 76.4 to 84.4.

d.   *What is the gain from stratified random sampling over what would have been obtained from simple random sampling?*

Solution: In this example, there is no gain from stratified sampling. This is likely due to the fact that employees in exposure category 1 had quite different *fvc* measures. If there had been optimal allocation, then a greater number of individuals would have been sampled from this stratum, and the estimate would have been better than that obtained from simple random sampling.

6.3   *Let us suppose that a household survey is to be taken for the purpose of estimating characteristics of families having female household heads. Since it is not known in advance of the survey which families have female household heads, the sample households will be screened and those sample households with female heads will be given a detailed interview. It is anticipated that the cost of screening a household is $10.00 and of interviewing a household having a female head is $50.00. The population is stratified into three strata according to the latest census information on the proportion of households having female heads. The strata are shown in the accompanying table. Assume that the variance of the characteristics being measured is the same in each stratum and that a total budget of $10,000 is allowed for the fieldwork. How many households in each stratum should be sampled?*

Stratum	No. of Households	Percentage of Households Having Female Head
1	10,000	25
2	20,000	15
3	5,000	10

Solution: Using equation 6.19 on page 161 in the book:

$$n_h = \left(\frac{N_h \sigma_{hx} \Big/ \sqrt{C_h}}{\sum_{h=1}^{L} N_h \sigma_{hx} \sqrt{C_h}} \right) * C$$

$C = \$10,000$
$C_1 = \$10 + 0.25 * \$50 = \$22.50, \ N_1 = 10,000$
$C_2 = \$10 + 0.15 * \$50 = \$17.50, \ N_2 = 20,000$
$C_3 = \$10 + 0.10 * \$50 = \$15.00, \ N_3 = 5,000$

$$n_1 = \frac{10,000 \div \sqrt{22.50}}{\left(10,000 * \sqrt{22.50}\right) + \left(20,000 * \sqrt{17.50}\right) + \left(5,000 * \sqrt{15.00}\right)} * 10,000$$
$$= 140.11 \approx 140$$

$$n_2 = \frac{20,000 \div \sqrt{17.50}}{\left(10,000 * \sqrt{22.50}\right) + \left(20,000 * \sqrt{17.50}\right) + \left(5,000 * \sqrt{15.00}\right)} * 10,000$$
$$= 317.74 \approx 318$$

$$n_3 = \frac{5,000 \div \sqrt{15.00}}{\left(10,000 * \sqrt{22.50}\right) + \left(20,000 * \sqrt{17.50}\right) + \left(5,000 * \sqrt{15.00}\right)} * 10,000$$
$$= 85.8 \approx 86$$

6.4   *Consider the 40 workers presented in Table 3.8 to be a simple random sample from the*
      1200 workers in the plant.

a.   *Compute a 90% confidence interval for the population mean forced vital capacity.*

      Solution: Using the survey procedures in STATA:

```
. gen N = 1200
. gen wt1 = N/40

. svyset _n [pweight=wt1], fpc(N)
      pweight: wt1
          VCE: linearized
  Single unit: missing
     Strata 1: <one>
        SU 1: <observations>
       FPC 1: N

. svy: mean fvc, level(90)
(running mean on estimation sample)

Survey: Mean estimation

Number of strata =         1         Number of obs    =        40
Number of PSUs   =        40         Population size  =      1200
                                     Design df        =        39


-----------------------------------------------------------------
                 |            Linearized
                 |    Mean    Std. Err.    [90% Conf. Interval]
-----------------+-----------------------------------------------
           fvc |    80.4    1.928777      77.15025    83.64975
-----------------------------------------------------------------
```

      The 90% confidence interval for the population mean forced vital capacity is 77.2 to
      83.6.

b.   *Suppose it is known, prior to analyzing the data, that the 1200 workers were distributed as follows:*

$N_1 = 100$ *(number with low exposure)*
$N_2 = 100$ *(number with medium exposure)*
$N_3 = 1000$ *(number with high exposure)*

Poststratify the original sample of Table 3.8 and construct a 90% confidence interval for the population mean forced vital capacity

Solution: We will use the formulas on pages 169 and 170 in the book to obtain the poststratified mean and variance.

$$\bar{x}_{pstr} = \sum_{h=1}^{L} \left(\frac{N_h}{N}\right) \bar{x}_h$$

$$\widehat{Var}(\bar{x}_{pstr}) = \left(\frac{N-n}{nN}\right) \sum_{h=1}^{L} \left(\frac{N_h}{N}\right) s_{hx}^2 + \left(\frac{1}{n^2}\right) \sum_{h=1}^{L} s_{hx}^2 \left(\frac{N-n_h}{N}\right)$$

Next, we will use STATA to calculate the mean variance of the FVC, for each level of exposure.

```
. bysort exposure: sum fvc

------------------------------------------------------------------------------
    > exposure = 1

    Variable |      Obs        Mean     Std. Dev.        Min         Max
-------------+----------------------------------------------------------
         fvc |        6    83.33333     13.9523          64          99

------------------------------------------------------------------------------
-> exposure = 2

    Variable |      Obs        Mean     Std. Dev.        Min         Max
-------------+----------------------------------------------------------
         fvc |        6        83.5      11.077          70          99

------------------------------------------------------------------------------
-> exposure = 3

    Variable |      Obs        Mean     Std. Dev.        Min         Max
-------------+----------------------------------------------------------
         fvc |       28    79.10714    12.56196          60          98
```

Applying the formulas, we get:

$$\bar{x}_{pstr} = \sum_{h=1}^{L}\left(\frac{N_h}{N}\right)\bar{x}_h = \left(\frac{100}{1200}\right)*83.33333 + \left(\frac{100}{1200}\right)*83.5 + \left(\frac{1000}{1200}\right)*79.10714$$
$$= 79.825$$

$$\widehat{Var}(\bar{x}_{pstr}) = \left(\frac{N-n}{nN}\right)\sum_{h=1}^{L}\left(\frac{N_h}{N}\right)s_{hx}^2 + \left(\frac{1}{n^2}\right)\sum_{h=1}^{L}s_{hx}^2\left(\frac{N-n_h}{N}\right)$$
$$= \left(\frac{1200-40}{40(1200)}\right)\left(\frac{100}{1200}*194.67 + \frac{100}{1200}*122.70 + \frac{1000}{1200}*157.80\right) + \frac{1}{40^2}$$
$$* \left(\frac{1200-6}{1200}*194.67 + \frac{1200-6}{1200}*122.70 + \frac{1200-28}{1200}*157.80\right) = 4.1108$$

$$\widehat{SE}(\bar{x}_{pstr}) = \sqrt{4.1108} = 2.028$$

The approximate 90% confidence interval after poststratifying the sample is:

$$79.825 \pm 1.645(2.028) = 79.825 \pm 3.336 = (76.489, 83.161)$$

Using the survey procedures in STATA:

```
. gen postwt=100
. replace postwt=1000 if exposure==3
(6 real changes made)

. svyset _n [pweight=wt1], fpc(N1) poststrata(exposure) postweight(postwt)

      pweight: wt1
          VCE: linearized
   Poststrata: exposure
   Postweight: postwt
  Single unit: missing
     Strata 1: <one>
        SU 1: <observations>
       FPC 1: N1

. svy: mean fvc, level(90)
(running mean on estimation sample)

Survey: Mean estimation

Number of strata =        1      Number of obs   =      40
Number of PSUs   =       40      Population size =    1200
N. of poststrata =        3      Design df       =      39

--------------------------------------------------------------
             |             Linearized
             |     Mean    Std. Err.    [90% Conf. Interval]
-------------+------------------------------------------------
         fvc |  79.8254    2.011272     76.43665     83.21414
--------------------------------------------------------------
```

c.   *Compare the intervals of parts (a) and (b). Which is larger? Why?*

Solution: The poststratified interval is slightly wider than the one obtained assuming simple random sampling. Poststratification results in a more efficient estimate only when the strata are homogeneous with respect to the variable of interest. In this example, the strata, exposure levels, are not homogeneous. The FVC values are not greatly different as exposure level increases. There is overlap between the strata and the point estimates for strata 1 and 2 are very similar. Thus, there is no benefit in using the additional information about the strata sizes.

6.5   *A marketing research firm specializing in the health care industry has a file containing approximately 150,000,000 names organized by zip codes (the file contains 65,000 zip codes). A stratified random sample is to be taken with zip codes as the strata and proportional allocation. The purpose of this survey is to estimate the proportion of persons who would be likely to purchase a new type of electric toothbrush. An intensive marketing program would be initiated if, as a result of the survey, 15% or more of the population indicate willingness to purchase the product. How many names per zip code should be sampled if it is desired to estimate with 95% confidence this proportion to within 5% of its true value?*

Solution: Let $N = 150,000,000$, $z = 1.96$, $\varepsilon = 0.05$, and $P = 0.15$. Using equation 6.24 on page 176, we get:

$$n \approx \frac{N z^2_{1-(\alpha/2)} * \left(\sigma^2_{wx}/\bar{x}^2\right)}{z^2_{1-(\alpha/2)} * \left(\sigma^2_{wx}/\bar{x}^2\right) + N\varepsilon^2}$$

We will assume that $\sigma^2_{wx} = (0.15)(0.85) = 0.1275$ *and* $\bar{X} = 0.15$.

$$n \approx \frac{150,000,000 * 1.96^2 * \left(\frac{0.1275}{0.15^2}\right)}{1.96^2 * \left(\frac{0.1275}{0.15^2}\right) + 150,000,000 * 0.05^2} = 8707.1 \ or \ 8708$$

8707.1/65,000 = 0.134 per zip code. Thus, 1 household per zip code would more than meet specifications.

6.6   *Esther is an epidemiologist and a very successful amateur body builder ("Ms. Drug Free Chicago Upper Body, 2000"). She is planning a survey of Chicago area body builders to determine the proportion who have ever used anabolic steroids. Her sampling frame consists of membership lists obtained from all accredited health clubs in the six-county Chicago metropolitan area. She has stratified clubs into the following three groups on the basis of their clientele:*

1. *Inner city yuppie*
2. *Inner city blue collar*
3. *Suburban*

She anticipates that the proportion using anabolic steroids will be twice as high in stratum 1, which contains most of the "hard-core" competitors as in stratum 2, and that the proportion in stratum 3 will be about two-thirds as high as that in stratum 2. From her membership lists, she enumerates 8345 members in stratum 1, 5286 in stratum 2, and 6300 in stratum 3. If she can sample 1000 persons, how many should be allocated to each stratum? (Assume overall proportion using steroids is 12%.)

Solution: In optimal allocation, the sample is allocated so that the estimates that result have the lowest variance among all possible ways of allocating the total sample.

Let P_2 be the proportion of individuals using steroids in stratum 2, $P_3 = 2/3*P_2$, and $P_1 = 2P_2$.

We can solve for P_2 and then find P_1 and P_3. Once we have these values we can find the variances and solve for the n's.

$$8345(2 * P_2) + 5286(P_2) + 6300\left(\frac{2}{3}P_2\right) = 19{,}931(0.12)$$

$$P_2(16{,}690 + 5286 + 4200) = 2391.72$$

$$P_2 = 0.0914; \ P_1 = 0.1827; \ P_3 = 0.0609$$

$$\sigma_1 = [P_1(1 - P_1)]^{1/2} = [0.1827(1 - 0.1827)]^{1/2} = 0.3864$$

$$\sigma_2 = [P_2(1 - P_2)]^{1/2} = [0.0914(1 - 0.0914)]^{1/2} = 0.2882$$

$$\sigma_3 = [P_3(1 - P_3)]^{1/2} = [0.0609(1 - 0.0609)]^{1/2} = 0.2391$$

$$n_1 = \frac{N_1\sigma_1}{N_1\sigma_1 + N_2\sigma_2 + N_3\sigma_3} * 1000$$

$$= \frac{8345 * 0.3864}{8345 * 0.3864 + 5286 * 0.2882 + 6300 * 0.2391} * 1000 = 515.6 \; or \; 516$$

$$n_2 = \frac{N_2\sigma_2}{N_1\sigma_1 + N_2\sigma_2 + N_3\sigma_3} * 1000 = \frac{1523.425}{6254.263} * 1000 = 243.58 \; or \; 244$$

$$n_3 = \frac{N_3\sigma_3}{N_1\sigma_1 + N_2\sigma_2 + N_3\sigma_3} * 1000 = \frac{1506.33}{6254.263} * 1000 = 240.8 \; or \; 241$$

6.7   *Esther (the heroine of Exercise 6.6) is able to obtain $25,000 from BBAAS (Body Builders Against Anabolic Steroids) to conduct her survey. This will be her only source of funding. She estimates that it would cost $30.00 per interview in strata 1 and 2, and $40.00 per interview in stratum 3. With this in mind, how many persons should she interview in each stratum?*

Solution: In this problem, the total cost is fixed at $25,000. We therefore need to use the equation for optimal allocation when the cost is fixed, which is equation 6.19 in the book. We will use the information that was calculated for Exercise 6.6. Let us assume that $\sigma_1 = 0.3864$, $\sigma_2 = 0.2882$, and $\sigma_3 = 0.2391$.

$$n_1 = \frac{8345(0.3864) \div \sqrt{30}}{8345(0.3864) \div \sqrt{30} + 5286(0.2882) \div \sqrt{30} + 6300(0.2391) \div \sqrt{30}} * \$25,000 \approx 414$$

$$n_2 = \frac{5286(0.2882) \div \sqrt{30}}{8345(0.3864) \div \sqrt{30} + 5286(0.2882) \div \sqrt{30} + 6300(0.2391) \div \sqrt{30}} * \$25,000 \approx 196$$

$$n_3 = \frac{6300(0.2391) \div \sqrt{30}}{8345(0.3864) \div \sqrt{30} + 5286(0.2882) \div \sqrt{30} + 6300(0.2391) \div \sqrt{30}} * \$25,000 \approx 168$$

Total Cost = 414($30) + 196($30) + 168($40) = $25,020

6.8   *Esther (the same Esther from Exercises 6.6 and 6.7) feels that it would only be worthwhile to do her survey if she can be 95% certain of estimating the rate to within 15% of its true value. She anticipates that the true overall rate will be about 12%. Based on her funding level indicated in Exercise 6.7, does she have enough funds to meet her specifications?*

Solution: We must first calculate a sample size using equation 6.24 on page 176.

$$n \approx \frac{N z^2_{1-(\alpha/2)} * \left(\sigma^2_{wx} / \bar{x}^2\right)}{z^2_{1-(\alpha/2)} * \left(\sigma^2_{wx} / \bar{x}^2\right) + N\varepsilon^2}$$

We will assume that $\sigma^2_{wx} = (0.12)(0.88) = 0.1056$ *and* $\bar{X} = 0.12$.

$$n \approx \frac{19{,}931 * 1.96^2 * \left(\frac{0.1056}{0.12^2}\right)}{19{,}931 * 0.15^2 + 1.96^2 * \left(\frac{0.1056}{0.12^2}\right)} = \frac{561{,}490.817}{448.4475 + 28.1717} = 1178.1 \ or \ 1179$$

Next, we will allocate the 1179 people to the three strata using optimal allocation, equation 6.18 on page 161.

$$n_1 = \frac{8345(0.3864) \div \sqrt{30}}{8345(0.3864) \div \sqrt{30} + 5286(0.2882) \div \sqrt{30} + 6300(0.2391) \div \sqrt{30}} * 1179$$
$$\approx 628$$

$$n_2 = \frac{5286(0.2882) \div \sqrt{30}}{8345(0.3864) \div \sqrt{30} + 5286(0.2882) \div \sqrt{30} + 6300(0.2391) \div \sqrt{30}} * 1179$$
$$\approx 297$$

$$n_3 = \frac{6300(0.2391) \div \sqrt{30}}{8345(0.3864) \div \sqrt{30} + 5286(0.2882) \div \sqrt{30} + 6300(0.2391) \div \sqrt{30}} * 1179$$
$$\approx 254$$

Total Cost = 628($30) + 297($30) + 254($40) = $18,840 + $8910 + $10,160
= $37,910

No, Esther does not have enough money to conduct her survey if she wants to be 95% certain of estimating the rate to within 15%.

6.9   *In a large population survey, 15,000 persons were screened with chest radiographs. Physicians noted possible pulmonary artery enlargement in 230 of these patients. This enlargement was confirmed by a second reading in 203 of these 230 patients. A sample of 175 of the 14,770 chest radiographs in which no enlargement of the pulmonary artery was noted yielded 12 radiographs that were actually positive for pulmonary artery enlargement.*

a.   *Based on these data, what is the prevalence of pulmonary artery enlargement in the population?*

Solution: The prevalence in the population is a weighted average of the prevalence estimates from the two strata.

$$Prevalence = \frac{230\left(\frac{203}{230}\right) + 14{,}770(\frac{12}{175})}{15{,}000} = 0.081$$

b.   *Obtain 95% confidence intervals for this prevalence rate.*

Solution: Use equation 6.8 in Box 6.2 on page 149 in book to estimate the standard error.

$$\widehat{SE}(prev) = \sqrt{\sum_{h=1}^{L}\left(\frac{N_h}{N}\right)^2 \frac{p_{hy}(1-p_{hy})}{n_h-1}\left(\frac{N_h-n}{N_h}\right)}$$

$$= \sqrt{\left(\frac{230}{15{,}000}\right)\left(\frac{0.8826*0.1174}{229}\right)\left(\frac{0}{230}\right) + \left(\frac{14{,}770}{15{,}000}\right)\left(\frac{0.0686*0.9314}{174}\right)\left(\frac{14{,}595}{14{,}770}\right)}$$

$$= 0.0188$$

The 95% confidence interval for the prevalence rate is:

$$0.081 \pm 1.96(0.0188) = (0.044, 0.118)$$

6.10 *A marathon was conducted in a large city on September 3, 1989. Based on the entry applications, the following data were obtained.*

Age Group	N	Mean Number of Marathons Completed ($\bar{X}$)	Standard Deviation (σ_x)
≤30	2300	1.9	0.6
30-49	1478	2.3	0.8
50+	978	3.1	0.7

It is desired to take a sample of approximately 500 persons from this list for purposes of estimating the average number of miles run per week in preparation for this marathon. If we assumed that this might be proportional to the number of marathons completed, is there much to be gained by using a stratified random sample with proportional allocation over a simple random sample?

Solution: Stratified random sampling is superior to simple random sampling, in terms of variance reduction, when the stratum means are different. We can use equations 6.15 and 6.16 to determine if stratified random sampling should be used.

$$\sigma_{bx}^2 = \frac{\sum_{h=1}^L N_h(\bar{X}_h - \bar{X})^2}{N}$$

$$= \frac{2300(1.9 - 2.27)^2 + 1478(2.3 - 2.27)^2 + 978(3.1 - 2.27)^2}{4756}$$

$$= \frac{989.94}{4756} = 0.208$$

$$\sigma_{wx}^2 = \frac{\sum_{h=1}^L N_h \sigma_{hx}^2}{N} = \frac{2300(0.36) + 1478(0.64) + 978(0.49)}{4756} = 0.474$$

$$\frac{VAR(\bar{x})}{VAR(\bar{x}_{str})} = \frac{\sigma_{bx}^2 + \sigma_{wx}^2}{\sigma_{wx}^2} = 1 + \frac{\sigma_{bx}^2}{\sigma_{wx}^2} = 1 + \frac{0.208}{0.474} = 1.439$$

A 44% increase indicates that stratification will lead to a reduction in the variance of the estimated mean number of miles run per week in preparation for the marathon.

6.11   *This exercise relates to the illustrative example on screening for twins discussed in Section 6.5. White female-female pairs were constructed as described in the illustrative example on the basis of same date of birth and SS#'s matching on the first seven digits. The number of pairs so constructed is as follows:*

Quartile Based on SS # Sequence Difference	Number of Pairs Constructed from Medicare Files
First Quartile	10,024
Middle Two Quartiles	20,031
Fourth Quartile	10,024

Suppose that you guess that the overall prevalence of twins among these pairs is 20%, and that the prevalence of twins in the first quartile is twice that in the second quartile, while it is 3 times that in the third quartile. If you are planning to take a stratified random sample of 300 pairs from this file for the purposes of estimating the prevalence of twins in this file, what would be the optimal allocation in each of the three quartiles?

Solution: We must first solve for p_1 and then we can compute p_2 and p_3.

$$\frac{N_1 p_1 + N_2 p_1 \frac{1}{2} + N_3 p_1 \frac{1}{3}}{N} = 0.20$$

$$p_1 = 0.343, \qquad p_2 = 0.172, \qquad p_3 = 0.114$$

Next, we use these prevalence estimates in equation 6.17 to obtain the sample sizes for each stratum.

$$n_h = \left(\frac{N_h \sigma_{hx}}{\sum_{h=1}^{L} N_h \sigma_{hx}}\right)(n)$$

$$n_1 = \frac{(10{,}024\sqrt{0.343 * 0.657})}{(10{,}024\sqrt{0.343 * 0.657}) + (20{,}031\sqrt{0.172 * 0.828}) + (10{,}024\sqrt{0.114 * 0.886})}$$
$$* 300 = 92.2 \approx 92$$

$$n_2 = \frac{(20{,}031\sqrt{0.172 * 0.828})}{(10{,}024\sqrt{0.343 * 0.657}) + (20{,}031\sqrt{0.172 * 0.828}) + (10{,}024\sqrt{0.114 * 0.886})}$$
$$* 300 = 146.3 \approx 146$$

$$n_3 = \frac{(10{,}024\sqrt{0.114 * 0.886})}{(10{,}024\sqrt{0.343 * 0.657}) + (20{,}031\sqrt{0.172 * 0.828}) + (10{,}024\sqrt{0.114 * 0.886})}$$
$$* 300 = 61.6 \approx 62$$

Suppose that instead of a stratified random sample of 300 pairs, it is decided to take a simple random sample of 300 pairs and the following data are obtained:

Quartile Based on SS # Sequence Difference	Number of Pairs Sampled	Number of Twins
First Quartile	90	40
Middle Two Quartiles	110	10
Fourth Quartile	100	1

a. *What is the estimated prevalence of twins and its standard error?*

Solution: We will use the equations presented in Chapter 3 to obtain these estimates.

$$\hat{p} = \frac{51}{300} = 0.17$$

$$\widehat{SE}(\hat{p}) = \sqrt{\frac{N-n}{N}} \sqrt{\frac{\hat{p}(1-\hat{p})}{n-1}} = \sqrt{\frac{39{,}779}{40{,}079}} \sqrt{\frac{0.17(0.83)}{299}} = 0.0216$$

b. *Find the poststratified estimate of the prevalence of twins and its standard error.*

Solution: We will use the equations on pages 169 and 170 in the book to compute these estimates.

$$\hat{p}_{str} = \sum_{h=1}^{L} \left(\frac{N_h}{N}\right) \hat{p}_h$$

$$\widehat{Var}(\hat{p}_{str}) = \left(\frac{N-n}{nN}\right) \sum_{h=1}^{L} \frac{N_h}{N} s_{hx}^2 + \left(\frac{1}{n^2}\right) \sum_{h=1}^{L} s_{hx}^2 \left(\frac{N-n_h}{N}\right)$$

Applying the formulas to the data gives us:

$$\hat{p}_{str} = \sum_{h=1}^{L} \left(\frac{N_h}{N}\right) \hat{p}_h = \left(\frac{10{,}024}{40{,}079}\right) * 0.444 + \left(\frac{22{,}031}{40{,}079}\right) * 0.091 + \left(\frac{10{,}024}{40{,}079}\right) * 0.01$$
$$= 0.1815$$

$$\widehat{Var}(\hat{p}_{str}) = \left(\frac{N-n}{nN}\right) \sum_{h=1}^{L} \frac{N_h}{N} s_{hx}^2 + \left(\frac{1}{n^2}\right) \sum_{h=1}^{L} s_{hx}^2 \left(\frac{N-n_h}{N}\right)$$

$$= \left(\frac{40{,}079 - 300}{300(40{,}079)}\right) \left[\frac{10{,}024}{40{,}079} * (0.556 * 0.444) + \frac{20{,}031}{40{,}079}\right.$$

$$* (0.091 * 0.909) + \frac{10{,}024}{40{,}079} * (0.01 * 0.99)\Big]$$

$$+ \frac{1}{300^2} \left[\frac{40{,}079 - 10{,}024}{40{,}079} * (0.556 * 0.444) + \frac{40{,}079 - 20{,}031}{40{,}079}\right.$$

$$* (0.091 * 0.909) + \frac{40{,}079 - 10{,}024}{40{,}079} * (001 * 0.99)\Big]$$

$$= 0.00362 + 0.000002596 = 0.0003646$$

$$SE(\hat{p}_{str}) = \sqrt{0.0003646} = 0.0191$$

Chapter Seven – Solutions

7.1   *A sample survey is being planned in which it is desired to estimate the average ratio of medical expenses to family income in a large city containing 234,785 families. Based on data in the table accompanying Exercise 7.2, how many families would have to be sampled if it is desired to estimate with 95% certainty this parameter to within 5% of its true value?*

Solution: *Equation 7.13 will be used to estimate this sample size. The data in the table accompanying Exercise 7.2 will be used as preliminary data in the sample size calculation.*

```
. list

        fam_id   fam_size    income    med_exp
  1.        1          2        372       28.6
  2.        2          3        372       41.6
  3.        3          3        522       45.4
  4.        4          5        390         61
  5.        5          4        348       82.4
  6.        6          7        552       56.4
  7.        7          2        528       48.4
  8.        8          4        574         60
  9.        9          2        498       48.4
 10.       10          5        372       88.8
 11.       11          3        378       26.8
 12.       12          6        372       39.6
 13.       13          4        360       58.8
 14.       14          4        450       54.2
 15.       15          2        540       44.2
 16.       16          5        450       75.4
 17.       17          3        414       45.2
 18.       18          4        498         72
 19.       19          2        510       21.2
 20.       20          4        438       55.4
 21.       21          2        396       51.9
 22.       22          5        348       46.6
 23.       23          3        462       79.6
 24.       24          4        414       33.6
 25.       25          7        390       75.6
 26.       26          3        462       69.6
 27.       27          3        414       57.4
 28.       28          6        570        126
 29.       29          2        462       39.1
 30.       30          2        414       43.2
 31.       31          6        414       36.4
 32.       32          4        402       40.2
 33.       33          2        378       41.4
```

```
. sum income med_exp, detail

                              income
-------------------------------------------------------------
        Percentiles     Smallest
 1%          348            348
 5%          348            348
10%          372            360          Obs                  33
25%          378            372          Sum of Wgt.          33

50%          414                         Mean            438.303
                         Largest         Std. Dev.      67.62234
75%          498            540
90%          540            552          Variance        4572.78
95%          570            570          Skewness       .5615178
99%          574            574          Kurtosis       2.115228

                             med_exp
-------------------------------------------------------------
        Percentiles     Smallest
 1%         21.2           21.2
 5%         26.8           26.8
10%         33.6           28.6          Obs                  33
25%         41.4           33.6          Sum of Wgt.          33

50%         48.4                         Mean            54.37576
                         Largest         Std. Dev.      20.97364
75%           61           79.6
90%         79.6           82.4          Variance       439.8938
95%         88.8           88.8          Skewness       1.260912
99%          126            126          Kurtosis       5.339344


. corr income med_exp
(obs=33)

             |   income  med_exp
-------------+------------------
     income  |   1.0000
    med_exp  |   0.2076   1.0000
```

To estimate the sample size, let N = 234,785, ε = 0.05.

$$n = \frac{z_{1-\alpha/2}^2 * N * (V_x^2 + V_y^2 - 2\rho_{xy}V_xV_y)}{z_{1-\alpha/2}^2 * (V_x^2 + V_y^2 - 2\rho_{xy}V_xV_y) + (N-1)\varepsilon^2}$$

$$\hat{V}_x^2 = \left(\frac{N-1}{N}\right)\left(\frac{s_x^2}{\bar{x}^2}\right) = \left(\frac{2699}{2700}\right)\left(\frac{439.89}{54.38^2}\right) = 0.149$$

$$\hat{V}_y^2 = \left(\frac{N-1}{N}\right)\left(\frac{s_y^2}{\bar{y}^2}\right) = \left(\frac{2699}{2700}\right)\left(\frac{4572.78}{438.30^2}\right) = 0.024$$

$$\hat{\rho}_{xy} = 0.2076$$

$$n = \frac{1.96^2 * 234{,}785 * [0.149 + 0.024 - 2(0.2076)(0.386)(0.155)]}{1.96^2 * [0.149 + 0.024 - 2(0.2076)(0.386)(0.155)] + 234{,}784 * 0.05^2}$$
$$= 227.39 \ or \ 228$$

7.2   *The accompanying table, based on a simple random sample of 33 families from a community of 600 families, gives the family size, weekly net family income, and weekly cost of medical expenditures including pharmaceuticals. The community contains 2700 persons.*

a.   *Estimate and give a 95% confidence interval for the average weekly medical expenditure per family.*

> ***Solution:*** *Using Stata, the mean weekly medical expenditure per family can be estimated.*

```
. gen N = 600

. gen wt = N / 33

. svyset _n [pweight=wt], fpc(N)

      pweight: wt
          VCE: linearized
  Single unit: missing
     Strata 1: <one>
         SU 1: <observations>
        FPC 1: N

. svy: mean med_exp
(running mean on estimation sample)

Survey: Mean estimation

Number of strata =        1      Number of obs   =       33
Number of PSUs   =       33      Population size =      600
                                 Design df       =       32

--------------------------------------------------------------
             |                 Linearized
             |      Mean     Std. Err.     [95% Conf. Interval]
-------------+------------------------------------------------
     med_exp |   54.37576   3.549219       47.14623    61.60528
--------------------------------------------------------------
```

The average weekly medical expenditure per family is estimated to be $54.38 and a 95% confidence interval for this estimate is $47.15 to $61.61.

b. *Estimate and give a 95% confidence interval for the average weekly medical expenditure per person. Justify you method of estimation.*

Solution: *A ratio estimate will be used to approximate the average weekly medical expenditure per person because both the numerator and denominator are subject to sampling variation.*

```
. svy: ratio  med_exp  fam_size
(running ratio on estimation sample)

Survey: Ratio estimation

Number of strata =        1        Number of obs   =       33
Number of PSUs   =       33        Population size =      600
                                   Design df       =       32

     _ratio_1: med_exp/fam_size

-------------------------------------------------------------
            |                Linearized
            |      Ratio   Std. Err.     [95% Conf. Interval]
------------+------------------------------------------------
    _ratio_1 |   14.58862    1.029044     12.49252    16.68471
-------------------------------------------------------------
```

The estimated average weekly medical expenditure per person is $14.59 and the 95% confidence interval for this estimate is $12.49 to $16.68.

c.   *Estimate and give a 95% confidence interval for the average proportion of family income spent on medical expenses.*

      Solution: *Ratio estimation will be used for this problem.*

```
. svy: ratio  med_exp  income
(running ratio on estimation sample)

Survey: Ratio estimation

Number of strata =          1       Number of obs    =      33
Number of PSUs   =         33       Population size  =     600
                                    Design df        =      32

      _ratio_1: med_exp/income

----------------------------------------------------------------
               |                Linearized
               |     Ratio    Std. Err.    [95% Conf. Interval]
---------------+------------------------------------------------
      _ratio_1 |   .1240597     .008073     .1076156    .1405039
----------------------------------------------------------------
```

The average proportion of family income spent on medical expenses is 0.12 and a 95% confidence interval for this estimate is 0.11 to 0.14.

d. *Estimate and give a 95% confidence interval for the total weekly medical expenses paid by the community.*

Solution: *There are two ways to approach this problem. One is to use the simple inflation estimate that was presented in Chapter 3. The second approach involves ratio estimation of totals. In this problem, we have the estimates x', y' and Y. Thus, we can use all of this information to obtain a better estimate of the total weekly medical expenses.*

```
. gen med_exp1 = med_exp * 2700

. svy: ratio  med_exp1 fam_size
(running ratio on estimation sample)

Survey: Ratio estimation

Number of strata =          1       Number of obs    =        33
Number of PSUs   =         33       Population size  =       600
                                    Design df        =        32


      _ratio_1: med_exp1/fam_size

-----------------------------------------------------------------
             |              Linearized
             |      Ratio   Std. Err.     [95% Conf. Interval]
-------------+---------------------------------------------------
    _ratio_1 |   39389.27   2778.418      33729.82     45048.72
-----------------------------------------------------------------
```

The ratio estimated total weekly medical expenses paid by the community is $39,389.27 and a 95% confidence interval for this estimate is $33,729.82 to $45048.72.

```
. svy: total  med_exp
(running total on estimation sample)

Survey: Total estimation

Number of strata =          1       Number of obs    =        33
Number of PSUs   =         33       Population size  =       600
                                    Design df        =        32


-----------------------------------------------------------------
             |              Linearized
             |      Total   Std. Err.     [95% Conf. Interval]
-------------+---------------------------------------------------
     med_exp |   32625.45   2129.532      28287.74     36963.17
-----------------------------------------------------------------
```

The inflation estimate of the total is $32,625.45, which is less than the ratio estimate of the total.

e.   *Estimate and give a 95% confidence interval for the average proportion of family income spent on medical expenses for families whose weekly net income is less than $400. Do the same for those whose weekly net income is greater than $400.*

     Solution: *A variable must be created that defines these two groups of families (i.e. those with a weekly income above $400 and those with an income below $400).*

```
. gen low_inc=(income<=400)

. tab low_inc

   low_inc |      Freq.      Percent        Cum.
-----------+-----------------------------------
         0 |         21        63.64       63.64
         1 |         12        36.36      100.00
-----------+-----------------------------------
     Total |         33       100.00

. sort low_inc

. svy: ratio  med_exp income, over( low_inc)
(running ratio on estimation sample)

Survey: Ratio estimation

Number of strata =          1      Number of obs    =      33
Number of PSUs   =         33      Population size  =     600
                                   Design df        =      32

     _ratio_1: med_exp/income

          0: low_inc = 0
          1: low_inc = 1


-----------------------------------------------------------------
           |               Linearized
      Over |      Ratio    Std. Err.     [95% Conf. Interval]
-----------+-----------------------------------------------------
_ratio_1   |
         0 |   .1152683    .0090383      .0968579    .1336787
         1 |   .1436774    .0150664      .1129881    .1743667
-----------------------------------------------------------------
```

The proportion of family income spent on medical expenses for families whose weekly income is below $400 is 0.14 and the 95% confidence interval is 0.11 to 0.17. The proportion for families with a weekly income above $400 is 0.12 and the 95% confidence interval is 0.10 to 0.13. We see that families with a lower income spend a greater proportion of the weekly income on medical expenses.

7.3   *For the city cited in Exercise 7.2, it is also desired to estimate with virtual certainty the total moneys spent on medical expenses to within 10% of its true value. How many families would have to be sampled if these specifications were to be met?*

Solution: *There are two ways in which the sample size can be calculated in this problem. You can assume that a simple inflation estimate will be used to estimate the total and then you would calculate a sample size assuming simple random sampling. Or, you can assume that a ratio estimate of the total will be used to estimate the total, which would require using the sample size formula presented in Chapter 7. We will examine both estimates below.*

If we assume that we are estimating X using the estimate x', then Equation 3.14 should be used.

$$n = \frac{z_{1-\alpha/2}^2 * N * V_x^2}{z_{1-\alpha/2}^2 * V_x^2 + (N-1) * \varepsilon^2} = \frac{9 * 600 * 0.149}{9 * 0.149 * 599 * 0.10^2} = \frac{804.6}{7.331}$$

$$= 109.5 \text{ or } 110$$

If, instead, we assume that we are using the estimate x'', then Equation 7.13 should be used.

$$n = \frac{z_{1-\alpha/2}^2 * N * (V_x^2 + V_y^2 - 2\rho_{xy}V_xV_y)}{z_{1-\alpha/2}^2 * (V_x^2 + V_y^2 - 2\rho_{xy}V_xV_y) + (N-1)\varepsilon^2}$$

From exercise 7.1, we know that:

$$\widehat{V_x^2} = \left(\frac{N-1}{N}\right)\left(\frac{s_x^2}{\bar{x}^2}\right) = \left(\frac{2699}{2700}\right)\left(\frac{439.89}{54.38^2}\right) = 0.149$$

We must calculate:

$$\widehat{V_y^2} = \left(\frac{N-1}{N}\right)\left(\frac{s_y^2}{\bar{y}^2}\right) \text{ and } \hat{\rho}_{xy}$$

Using STATA, we get:

```
. sum fam_size, detail

                            fam_size
-------------------------------------------------------------
      Percentiles      Smallest
 1%        2               2
 5%        2               2
10%        2               2         Obs                   33
25%        2               2         Sum of Wgt.           33

50%        4                         Mean            3.727273
                       Largest       Std. Dev.       1.526285
75%        5               6
90%        6               6         Variance        2.329545
95%        7               7         Skewness        .5771234
99%        7               7         Kurtosis        2.387775

. corr fam_size med_exp
(obs=33)

             | fam_size  med_exp
-------------+------------------
    fam_size |   1.0000
     med_exp |   0.4518    1.0000
```

$$\hat{V}_y^2 = \left(\frac{N-1}{N}\right)\left(\frac{s_y^2}{\bar{y}^2}\right) = \left(\frac{599}{600}\right)\left(\frac{2.3295}{3.7273^2}\right) = 0.167$$

$$\hat{\rho}_{xy} = 0.4518$$

$$n = \frac{(*\,600*[0.149 + 0.167 - 2(0.4518)(0.386)(0.409)]}{9*[0.149 + 0.167 - 2(0.4518)(0.386)(0.409)] + 599*0.10^2}$$

$$= \frac{938.059}{1.563 + 5.99} = 124.19 \; or \; 125$$

7.4   *For the data in the table accompanying Exercise 7.2, obtain a regression estimate of the total weekly medical expenditures paid by the community. Give 95% confidence intervals for the true value of this parameter based on this regression line.*

         Solution: *To obtain a regression estimate of the total weekly medical expenditures, we will use equation 7.14 in the book.*

$$x'' = x' + b(Y - y')$$

STATA can be used to obtain x', y' *and* b.

```
. svy: total  med_exp
(running total on estimation sample)

Survey: Total estimation

Number of strata =          1      Number of obs    =        33
Number of PSUs   =         33      Population size  =       600
                                   Design df        =        32


----------------------------------------------------------------
               |                Linearized
               |     Total     Std. Err.     [95% Conf. Interval]
---------------+------------------------------------------------
      med_exp  |   32625.45     2129.532      28287.74    36963.17
----------------------------------------------------------------
. svy: total  fam_size
(running total on estimation sample)

Survey: Total estimation

Number of strata =          1      Number of obs    =        33
Number of PSUs   =         33      Population size  =       600
                                   Design df        =        32


--------------------------------------------------------------
               |                Linearized
               |     Total     Std. Err.     [95% Conf. Interval]
---------------+----------------------------------------------
     fam_size  |   2236.364     154.9693      1920.701     2552.026
--------------------------------------------------------------
```

```
. corr med_exp fam_size
(obs=33)

               |  med_exp fam_size
---------------+------------------
      med_exp  |   1.0000
     fam_size  |   0.4518   1.0000

. display 0.4518*(2129.532/154.9693)
6.208472
```

The regression estimate of the total and the standard error of this estimate are the following:

```
. display 32625.45 + 6.208472*(2700-2236.364)
35503.921

. display sqrt((2129.532^2) * (1 - 0.4518^2))
1899.7965
```

The 95% confidence interval is $35,503.92 ± 1.96*1899.80 = $31,780.31 to $39,227.53.

7.5   *It is desired to estimate the total, X, of nurse practitioner hours spent in direct patient care in a large HMO during a given year. This is to be done by taking a simple random sample of patients, and determining for each visit during the year, the number of practitioner hours spent during the visit. It is known that there are 3524 members of the HMO and that 8950 visits took place during that year. A small pilot sample of 10 patients yielded the following data:*

Patient	Visits	Nurse Practitioner Hours
1	0	0
2	5	3
3	1	0
4	2	6
5	3	3
6	7	0
7	1	0
8	1	2
9	0	0
10	4	3

Based on these pilot data, would you recommend a simple inflation estimate or a ratio estimate as the estimation method for the sample survey? Document the reasons for your recommendation.

Solution: *We can use the methods outlined in Section 7.5 in the book to determine which estimate of the total is likely to be better. The ratio estimate of the total, x'', will have a smaller variance than the simple inflation estimate, x', whenever $V_y/V_x < 2\rho_{xy}$.*

```
. sum Visits RN_Hours, detail

                              Visits
-------------------------------------------------------------
        Percentiles      Smallest
  1%          0              0
  5%          0              0
 10%          0              1       Obs                 10
 25%          1              1       Sum of Wgt.         10

 50%         1.5                     Mean               2.4
                          Largest    Std. Dev.     2.319004
 75%          4              3
 90%          6              4       Variance      5.377778
 95%          7              5       Skewness      .7821187
 99%          7              7       Kurtosis      2.467523

                             RN_Hours
-------------------------------------------------------------
        Percentiles      Smallest
  1%          0              0
  5%          0              0
 10%          0              0       Obs                 10
 25%          0              0       Sum of Wgt.         10

 50%          1                      Mean               1.7
                          Largest    Std. Dev.     2.057507
 75%          3              3
 90%         4.5             3       Variance      4.233333
 95%          6              3       Skewness      .8277728
 99%          6              6       Kurtosis      2.701945

. corr  Visits RN_Hours
(obs=10)

             |    Visits RN_Hours
-------------+------------------
      Visits |    1.0000
    RN_Hours |    0.2142    1.0000
```

Vy and Vx can be obtained using the following equations:

```
. display sqrt((3523/3524)*5.3778/2.4^2)
.9661640

. display sqrt((3523/3524)*4.233/1.7^2)
1.210079
```

$$V_x/V_y = \frac{0.9662}{1.2101} - 0.7984$$

$$2\rho_{xy} = 0.4284$$

Because 0.7984 > 0.4284, the simple inflation estimate would be better.

7.6   *Based on the data in Exercise 7.5, how many patients would have to be sampled if a*
       simple inflation estimate were to be used?

Solution: *Equation 3.14 will be used to calculate the sample size. Let N = 3524, ε =*
0.10, and z = 1.96.

$$n = \frac{z_{1-\alpha/2}^2 * N * V_x^2}{z_{1-\alpha/2}^2 * V_x^2 + (N-1) * \varepsilon^2} = \frac{1.96^2 * 3524 * 1.2101^2}{1.96^2 * 1.2101^2 * 3523 * 0.10^2}$$

$$= \frac{19823.9669}{40.8554} = 485.22 \ or \ 486$$

7.7   *Based on the data in Exercise 7.5, how many patients would have to be sampled if a ratio*
       estimate were to be used?

Solution: *Equation 7.13 will be used to calculate the sample size. Let N = 3524, ε =*
0.10, and z = 1.96.

$$n = \frac{z_{1-\alpha/2}^2 * N * (V_x^2 + V_y^2 - 2\rho_{xy}V_xV_y)}{z_{1-\alpha/2}^2 * (V_x^2 + V_y^2 - 2\rho_{xy}V_xV_y) + (N-1)\varepsilon^2}$$

$$= \frac{1.96^2 * 3524 * [1.2101^2 + 0.9662^2 - 2(0.2142)(1.2101)(0.9662)]}{1.96^2 * [1.2101^2 + 0.9662^2 - 2(0.2142)(1.2101)(0.9662)] + 3523 * 0.10^2}$$

$$= \frac{25681.200}{42.5175} = 604.01 \ or \ 605$$

7.8   *A sample survey is to be conducted in which it is desired to estimate the proportion of persons over 70 years of age who have evidence of a cognitive impairment. This is to be done by taking a sample of households and giving a simple test of cognitive functioning to all members of the household over 70 years of age. A pilot study of 25 households yielded an average of 1.2 persons over 70 years of age per household with standard deviation equal to 0.8 and an average of 0.24 persons over 70 years of age per household showing evidence of cognitive impairment with standard deviation equal to 0.76. It is known that there are 3058 households in the community and 2949 persons over 70 years of age. How many households should be sampled if it is desired to estimate with 95% confidence the proportion of persons over 70 who show evidence of cognitive impairment within 20% of its true value?*

Solution: *Equation 7.13 will be used to calculate the sample size. Let N = 3058, ε = 0.20, and z = 1.96. The correlation coefficient, ρ_{xy} is not given, however we can use equation 7.10 to estimate it.*

$$n = \frac{z_{1-\alpha/2}^2 * N * (V_x^2 + V_y^2 - 2\rho_{xy}V_xV_y)}{z_{1-\alpha/2}^2 * (V_x^2 + V_y^2 - 2\rho_{xy}V_xV_y) + (N-1)\varepsilon^2}$$

$$\hat{V}_x^2 = \left(\frac{N-1}{N}\right)\left(\frac{s_x^2}{\bar{x}^2}\right) = \left(\frac{3057}{3058}\right)\left(\frac{0.76^2}{0.24^2}\right) = 10.024$$

$$\hat{V}_y^2 = \left(\frac{N-1}{N}\right)\left(\frac{s_y^2}{\bar{y}^2}\right) = \left(\frac{3057}{3058}\right)\left(\frac{0.80^2}{1.20^2}\right) = 0.444$$

$$\hat{\rho}_{xy} \approx \frac{\hat{V}_y}{\hat{V}_x} = \frac{0.667}{3.166} 0.2107$$

$$n = \frac{1.96^2 * 3058 * [10.024 + 0.444 - 2(0.2107)(3.166)(0.667)]}{1.96^2 * [10.024 + 0.444 - 2(0.2107)(3.166)(0.667)] + 3057 * 0.20^2}$$
$$= \frac{112520.05}{42.517159.08} = 707.3 \; or \; 708$$

7.9   *Show that for simple random sampling the correlation ρ_{xy} between two estimated totals x' and y' of characteristics X and Y is equal to ρ_{xy}, the correlation between X and Y.*

Solution:

The proof of this is very long and involved. It is outlined on page 57 in Hansen, Hurwitz and Madow, Volume 2 (1953).

7.10   *The following exercise was suggested by an article appearing in Public Health Reports [Petersen, LR, Dobb, R, and Dondero, TJ Jr. Methodological approaches to surveillance of HIV infection among blood donors. Public Health Reports 1990;105:153.]. A survey was taken to determine the incidence of HIV seroconversion among first-time blood donors at a blood center located in a large city. During a particular month, 180 first-time donors gave blood at the center. Of these, 175 were seronegative. A sample of 60 from the seronegative first-time donors was selected and given appointments to give blood again over the next 6 months. The following data were obtained from these persons.*

Months Since First Blood Donation	No. of Persons	HIV Status	
		Positive	Negative
3	18	2	16
4	10	2	8
5	8	1	7
6	7	0	7
7	6	2	4
8	5	0	5
9	4	1	3
10	2	1	1

From these data, estimate the annual incidence of HIV seroconversion among first-time blood donors at this center. Give a 95% confidence interval for this incidence rate.

Solution: *The incidence rate is defined as the number of new cases divided by the total person-time contribution over a specified time interval. We can use STATA to estimate the incidence rate and 95% confidence interval. First, the data have to be entered as a data set with 60 rows, one row per subject, and two variables, Month and Status.*

```
. list in 1/30

        month    status
  1.       3         1
  2.       3         1
  3.       3         0
  4.       3         0
  5.       3         0
  6.       3         0
  7.       3         0
  8.       3         0
  9.       3         0
 10.       3         0
 11.       3         0
 12.       3         0
 13.       3         0
 14.       3         0
 15.       3         0
 16.       3         0
 17.       3         0
 18.       3         0
 19.       4         1
 20.       4         1
 21.       4         0
 22.       4         0
 23.       4         0
 24.       4         0
 25.       4         0
 26.       4         0
 27.       4         0
 28.       4         0
 29.       5         1
 30.       5         0
```

Next, the svy: ratio procedure in STATA will be used to estimate the incidence rate and 95% confidence interval.

```
. gen N=175

. gen wt=N/60

. gen Years=month/12

. svyset _n [pweight=wt], fpc(N)
      pweight: wt
          VCE: linearized
  Single unit: missing
     Strata 1: <one>
         SU 1: <observations>
        FPC 1: N

. svy: ratio  status Years
(running ratio on estimation sample)

Survey: Ratio estimation

Number of strata =        1      Number of obs    =        60
Number of PSUs   =       60      Population size  =       175
                                 Design df        =        59

     _ratio_1: status/Years


------------------------------------------------------------
             |              Linearized
             |     Ratio   Std. Err.    [95% Conf. Interval]
-------------+----------------------------------------------
    _ratio_1 |   .343949   .0860694     .1717246    .5161735
------------------------------------------------------------
```

The estimated incidence rate per person-year is 0.34 and the 95% confidence interval is 0.17 to 0.52.

7.11   A large plant has 1000 workers. A simple random sample of 25 workers is taken to find the ratio of work-loss days to total days employed during the previous calendar year. The following data were obtained from the survey:

Total work-loss days among the 25 individuals sampled: 250
Total days employed among the 25 individuals sampled: 4375

a.   What is the estimated ratio of work-loss days to total days employed among workers in this plant?

Solution: The total work-loss days and total days employed, in the population of 1000 workers, have to be estimated first. Then, the ratio can be estimated.

$$x' = (1000/25)(250) = 10,000$$
$$y' = (1000/25)(4375) = 175,000$$
$$r = 10,000/175,000 = 0.05714$$

b.   *What further information would you need to estimate the standard error of this estimate?*

   Solution: *To estimate the standard error, we would need to know the distribution of the work loss days and days employed among the sampled workers because in the equation for the standard error, V_x, V_y, and ρ_{xy} must be known.*

c.   *From the information given above, estimate the total work-loss days among the 1000 workers in the cohort.*

   Solution: $x' = (1000/25)\,(250) = 10{,}000$

d.   *It so happens that the 1000 workers in the plant aggregate had 140,000 employment days during the previous calendar year. Based on this information, what would you infer about the estimate of total work-loss days computed in part (c)? Give reasons for your response.*

   Solution: *Y = total employment days among 1000 employees*
   y = total employment days among 25 employees in sample

$$x'' = rY = 0.05714(140{,}000) = 7999.6$$

The answer in part (c) is an overestimate. We used information obtained from the sample and this resulted in an estimate of 175,000 employment days. The true number of employment days is 140,000, which is much less than what we estimated with the sample. This therefore led to an overestimate of the total work-loss days.

7.12   *For the illustrative example in Section 7.3, suppose that the known number of hospitals in subdomain 1 is 50, and in subdomain 2 is 51.*

a.   *Determine the poststratified ratio estimate of the proportion of newborns discharged with the mother's hepatitis B surface antigen status documented on the newborn's record.*

Solution: *Using the equation for the poststratified ratio estimate in Section 7.3, we estimate:*

$$r_{pstr} = \frac{50/29 * 42,719 + 51/27 * 22,560}{50/29 * 47,850 + 51/27 * 38,929} = \frac{116,318.5}{156,032.6} = 0.745$$

b.   *Give reasons why this estimate is closer to the ordinary rate estimate than the poststratified estimate that was obtained in the illustrative example.*

Solution: *In this example, the subdomain ratio in the population is similar to the subdomain ratio in the sample. Thus, there is little gain when the true subdomain totals are applied in the poststratified estimate.*

Chapter Eight – Solutions

8.1   *Given a sample of 100 elements, which of the following designs is likely to yield estimates having the highest standard errors?*

   a. Systematic sampling
   b. Cluster sampling
   c. Simple random sampling
   d. Stratified random sampling

Solution: The answer is (b). Cluster sampling will result in an estimate that has the highest standard error.

8.2   *If one wished to sample this page for misspelled words, what would be a logical cluster?*

Solution: A logical cluster would be a paragraph. The listing unit would be the lines of text, and elementary units the words.

8.3   *If one wished to sample this entire book for misspelled words according to a three-stage cluster design, what could serve as primary sampling units, as secondary sampling units, as listing units, and as elementary units?*

Solution: The primary sampling unit would be the chapter. The secondary units would be the pages in each chapter. Lines of text would serve as the listing units, and words as the elementary units.

Chapter Nine – Solutions

9.1 *Suppose that the elementary schools in a city are grouped into 30 school districts, with each school district containing four schools. Suppose that a simple one-stage cluster sample of three school districts is taken for purposes of estimating the number of school children in the city who are color-blind (as measured by a standard test), and that the accompanying data are obtained from this sample. Estimate and obtain a 95% confidence interval for the total number of color-blind children and the proportion of all children who are color-blind.*

Sample School District	School	No. of Children	No. of Color-Blind Children
1	1	130	2
	2	150	3
	3	160	3
	4	120	5
2	1	110	2
	2	120	4
	3	100	0
	4	120	1
3	1	89	4
	2	130	2
	3	100	0
	4	150	2

Solution: We will use the equations contained in Box 9.2 in the book to estimate the total number of color-blind children and the proportion of all children who are color-blind, along with the 95% confidence intervals of these estimates.

Let $M = 30$, $m = 3$, and $N_i = 4$.

The estimated total number of color-blind children and 95% confidence interval are the following:

$$x'_{clu} = \left(\frac{M}{m}\right) x$$

$$x = \sum_{i=1}^{m} x_i = 28$$

$$\bar{x}_{clu} = \frac{x}{3} = \frac{28}{3} = 9.333$$

$$x'_{clu} = \left(\frac{30}{3}\right) 28 = 280$$

$$\widehat{SE}(x'_{clu}) = \frac{M}{\sqrt{m}} \sigma_{1x} \sqrt{\frac{M-m}{M-1}}$$

$$\hat{\sigma}_{1x} = \left[\frac{\sum_{i=1}^{m}(x_i - \bar{x}_{clu})^2}{m-1}\right]^{1/2} \sqrt{\frac{M-1}{M}}$$

$$\hat{\sigma}_{1x} = \left(\frac{13.4469 + 5.4429 + 1.7769}{2}\right)^{1/2} * 0.98319 = 3.1605$$

$$\widehat{SE}(x'_{clu}) = \frac{30}{\sqrt{3}} * 3.1605 * \sqrt{\frac{27}{29}} = 52.820$$

$$95\% \; CI = 280 \pm (1.96 * 52.82) = (176.5, 383.5)$$

Using STATA, we get the same estimated total and standard error, but a different confidence interval because STATA uses the t distribution to construct confidence intervals. In the hand calculations the standard normal distribution was used.

```
. gen M = 30
. gen wt = M / 3
. svyset  district [pweight=wt], fpc(M)
      pweight: wt
          VCE: linearized
  Single unit: missing
     Strata 1: <one>
         SU 1: district
        FPC 1: M

. svy: total  col_blnd
(running total on estimation sample)

Survey: Total estimation

Number of strata =          1        Number of obs   =        12
Number of PSUs   =          3        Population size =       120
                                     Design df       =         2

------------------------------------------------------------------
               |            Linearized
               |    Total   Std. Err.      [95% Conf. Interval]
---------------+--------------------------------------------------
      col_blnd |      280   52.82045      52.73194    507.2681
------------------------------------------------------------------
```

The estimated proportion of all children who are color-blind and the 95% confidence interval are the following:

$$r_{clu} = \frac{x}{y}$$

$$y = \sum_{i=1}^{m} y_i = 493$$

$$\bar{y}_{clu} = \frac{y}{m} = \frac{1479}{3} = 493$$

$$\widehat{SE}(r_{clu}) = r_{clu} \left\{ \frac{\left(\widehat{SE}(\bar{x}_{clu})\right)^2}{\bar{x}_{clu}^2} + \frac{\left(\widehat{SE}(\bar{y}_{clu})\right)^2}{\bar{y}_{clu}^2} - \frac{2}{m} * \frac{(M-m)}{M} * \frac{1}{\bar{x}_{clu}\bar{y}_{clu}} \right.$$
$$\left. * \frac{\sum_{i=1}^{m}(x_i - \bar{x}_{clu})(y_i - \bar{y}_{clu})}{m-1} \right\}^{1/2}$$

$$\widehat{SE}(\bar{x}_{clu}) = \frac{1}{\sqrt{m}} \sigma_{1x} \sqrt{\frac{M-m}{M-1}} = \frac{1}{\sqrt{3}} * 3.1605 * \sqrt{\frac{27}{29}} = 1.76$$

$$\widehat{SE}(\bar{y}_{clu}) = \frac{1}{\sqrt{m}} \sigma_{1y} \sqrt{\frac{M-m}{M-1}} = \frac{1}{\sqrt{3}} * 57.808 * \sqrt{\frac{27}{29}} = 32.205$$

$$\hat{\sigma}_{1y} = \left[\frac{\sum_{i=1}^{m}(y_i - \bar{y}_{clu})^2}{m-1} \right]^{1/2} \sqrt{\frac{M-1}{M}} = \left[\frac{4489 + 1849 + 576}{2} \right]^{1/2} \sqrt{\frac{29}{30}} = 57.808$$

$$\frac{\sum_{i=1}^{m}(x_i - \bar{x}_{clu})(y_i - \bar{y}_{clu})}{m-1}$$
$$= \frac{(13 - 9.333)(560 - 493) + (7 - 9.33)(450 - 493) + (8 - 9.333)(469 - 493)}{2} = 189$$

$$r_{clu} = \frac{28}{1479} = 0.019$$

$$\widehat{SE}(r_{clu}) = 0.019 \left\{ \frac{1.76^2}{9.33^2} + \frac{32.205^2}{493^2} - \frac{2}{3} * \left(\frac{27}{30}\right) * \left(\frac{1}{9.33 * 493}\right) * 189 \right\}^{1/2} = 0.00234$$

$$95\% \ CI = 0.019 \pm (1.96 * 0.00234) = (0.0144, 0.0236)$$

Using STATA, we get a similar ratio estimate and standard error, but again the confidence interval differs due to the fact that STATA uses a t distribution and we used a standard normal distribution in the calculation.

```
. svy: ratio  col_blnd   num_kids
(running ratio on estimation sample)

Survey: Ratio estimation

Number of strata =        1         Number of obs    =       12
Number of PSUs   =        3         Population size  =      120
                                    Design df        =        2


    _ratio_1: col_blnd/num_kids


-----------------------------------------------------------------
             |               Linearized
             |     Ratio    Std. Err.    [95% Conf. Interval]
-------------+---------------------------------------------------
    _ratio_1 |   .0189317    .0023347    .0088862     .0289772
-----------------------------------------------------------------
```

9.2   *A sample of patients is to be taken from the patient records of a large psychiatric outpatient clinic for purposes of estimating the total number of patients given tricyclic antidepressant drugs as part of their therapeutic regimen. The records are organized into file drawers, each containing 20 patient records, and there are 40 such file drawers.*

a.   *Suppose that we wish to use simple random sampling of patient records. How large a sample is needed if we wish to be virtually certain of estimating the total number of persons given tricyclic antidepressant drugs to within 10% of the true value and if we anticipate that approximately 20% of all patients were given these drugs?*

Solution: Assuming simple random sampling, we would use Equation 3.16, which is the sample size equation for estimating a proportion. We have to use this formula because there is not enough information to calculate a sample size for estimating a total, which requires an estimate of V_x.

$$n = \frac{z_{1-\alpha/2}^2 * N * P(1-P)}{z_{1-\alpha/2}^2 * P(1-P) + (N-1) * \varepsilon^2 * P^2} = \frac{9 * 800 * 0.2(0.8)}{9 * 0.2(0.8) + 799 * 0.10^2 * 0.2^2}$$

$$= \frac{1152}{1.7596} = 654.6 \; or \; 655$$

b. *What would be the field costs involved in taking the sample specified in part (a)? Make some assumptions about the cost components in determining these field costs.*

Solution: In this problem, we will assume that the total cost, C, is the sum of the costs associated with listing all 800 patients, C_0, and the cost for reviewing each of the 655 records in our sample, C_1. Thus, $C = C_0 + C_1$.

We can assume that it will cost 3 hours to list all 800 patients and 0.25 hour to review each record. The total cost is $C = 3 + (655*0.25) = 166.75$ hours.

c. *What sample size is needed if the design is to be a simple one-stage cluster sample [same specifications as in part (a)]?*

Solution: Assuming a one-stage sampling plan, we would use the sample size equation in Box 9.4.

$$m = \frac{z_{1-\alpha/2}^2 * M * P(1-P)}{z_{1-\alpha/2}^2 * P(1-P) + (M-1) * \varepsilon^2 * P^2} = \frac{9 * 40 * 0.2(0.8)}{9 * 0.2(0.8) + 39 * 0.10^2 * 0.2^2}$$

$$= \frac{57.6}{1.4556} = 39.6 \text{ or } 40$$

We would have to use all 40 clusters, and hence obtain information on the entire population.

d. *What would be the field costs for a simple one-stage cluster sample? Again, make some assumptions about the cost components in determining these field costs.*

Solution: In this problem, we will assume that the total cost, C, is the sum of the costs associated with enrolling the cluster into the study and constructing the sampling frame for that cluster (the costs that are not dependent on the number of enumeration units sampled) and the costs that can be expressed on a per-enumeration unit basis.

$$C = C_1 + C_2 mN = 3 + (0.25)(40)(20) = 203$$

As before, we will assume that 3 hours are required to construct the sampling frame (all clusters will have to be included) and 0.25 hour to review each record.

e. *Which of the two alternative sample designs would you use? Why?*

Solution: Because the simple random sampling plan would cost less to implement than the one-stage cluster sampling plan, it would be wise to choose simple random sampling. The reason it costs less is due to the fact that the entire population would have to be included in the one-stage cluster sample.

9.3   *A simple one-stage cluster sample was taken of 10 hospitals in a mid-western state from a population of 33 hospitals that have received state and federal funds to upgrade their emergency medical services. Within each of the hospitals selected in the sample, the records of all patients hospitalized in calendar year 1988 for traumatic injuries (i.e., accidents, poisonings, violence, burns, etc.) were examined. The number of patients hospitalized for trauma conditions and the number discharged dead are shown in the accompanying table for each hospital in the sample.*

Hospital	Total Number of Patients Hospitalized for Trauma Conditions	Total Number Discharged Dead Among All Patients Hospitalized with Trauma Conditions
1	560	4
2	190	4
3	260	2
4	370	4
5	190	4
6	130	0
7	170	9
8	170	2
9	60	0
10	110	1

a.   *For this sample, what are the clusters, what are the listing units, and what are the elementary units?*

Solution: The clusters are the hospitals, the listing units are the medical records for the patients hospitalized in 1988 for traumatic injuries, and the elementary units are the patients.

b.   *Estimate and give a 95% confidence interval for the total number of persons hospitalized for trauma conditions among the 33 hospitals.*

Solution: We can use STATA to obtain this estimate and 95% confidence interval. First, enter the data into the data editor.

```
. list tot_pat tot_dead

        tot_pat   tot_dead
  1.        560          4
  2.        190          4
  3.        260          2
  4.        370          4
  5.        190          4
  6.        130          0
  7.        170          9
  8.        170          2
  9.         60          0
 10.        110          1
```

Next, use the svy: total procedure to estimate the total number of persons hospitalized for trauma conditions.

```
. gen N = 33

. gen wt = N / 10

. svyset _n [pweight=wt], fpc(N)

      pweight: wt
          VCE: linearized
  Single unit: missing
     Strata 1: <one>
         SU 1: <observations>
        FPC 1: N

. svy: total  tot_pat
(running total on estimation sample)

Survey: Total estimation

Number of strata =        1        Number of obs     =       10
Number of PSUs   =       10        Population size   =       33
                                   Design df         =        9

-------------------------------------------------------------------
             |               Linearized
             |     Total    Std. Err.     [95% Conf. Interval]
-------------+-----------------------------------------------------
     tot_pat |      7293    1273.439      4412.282     10173.72
-------------------------------------------------------------------
```

The estimated number of persons hospitalized for trauma conditions among the 33 hospitals is 7923 and a 95% confidence interval for this estimate is 4412 to 10,174.

c.   *Estimate and give a 95% confidence interval for the total number of patients discharged dead among all persons hospitalized for trauma conditions.*

Solution: Again, we can use STATA to obtain this estimate and 95% confidence interval.

```
. svy: total  tot_dead
(running total on estimation sample)

Survey: Total estimation

Number of strata =         1      Number of obs   =       10
Number of PSUs   =        10      Population size =       33
                                  Design df       =        9


-----------------------------------------------------------------
             |               Linearized
             |      Total    Std. Err.     [95% Conf. Interval]
-------------+---------------------------------------------------
    tot_dead |         99    23.23216      46.4452     151.5548
-----------------------------------------------------------------
```

The estimated total number of patients discharged dead is 99 and the 95% confidence interval for this estimate is 46 to 152.

d.   *Estimate and give a 95% confidence interval for the proportion of patients discharged dead among those hospitalized with trauma conditions.*

Solution: We can use STATA to obtain this estimate and confidence interval.

```
. svy: ratio  tot_dead tot_pat
(running ratio on estimation sample)

Survey: Ratio estimation

Number of strata =         1      Number of obs   =       10
Number of PSUs   =        10      Population size =       33
                                  Design df       =        9

    _ratio_1: tot_dead/tot_pat

-----------------------------------------------------------------
             |               Linearized
             |      Ratio    Std. Err.     [95% Conf. Interval]
-------------+---------------------------------------------------
    _ratio_1 |   .0135747    .0033148      .0060761     .0210732
-----------------------------------------------------------------
```

The estimated proportion of patients discharged dead among those hospitalized with trauma conditions is 0.014 and the 95% confidence interval for this estimate is 0.006 to 0.021.

9.4   *The number of beds in each of the ten hospitals sampled in Exercise 9.3 is shown in the accompanying table. The remaining 23 hospitals not appearing in the sample have a total of 3687 beds. Use this information to obtain improved estimates and confidence intervals for the following:*

a.   *The total number of persons hospitalized with trauma conditions.*

b.   *The total number of persons discharged dead among all persons hospitalized with trauma conditions.*

Hospital	No. of Beds
1	824
2	312
3	329
4	648
5	358
6	252
7	256
8	263
9	138
10	150

Solution: We can compute a ratio estimate of the total number of persons hospitalized with trauma conditions. Let Z equal the total number of beds in the population, $Z = 3687 + 3530 = 7217$ and n equal the total in the sample, 3530.

Let Y = total number of persons hospitalized with trauma conditions and X = the total number of persons discharged dead.

$$y'' = y' * \frac{Z}{z'} = 2210 * \frac{7217}{3530} = 4518.3$$

$$\widehat{SE}(y'') = \frac{Z * r}{\sqrt{m}} (\hat{V}_y^2 + \hat{V}_z^2 - 2\hat{\rho}_{yz} \hat{V}_y \hat{V}_z)^{1/2} \sqrt{\frac{M-m}{M-1}}$$

$$\hat{\rho}_{yz} \approx \frac{\hat{V}_y}{\hat{V}_z}$$

$$\widehat{SE}(y'') = \frac{Z * r}{\sqrt{m}} (\hat{V}_y^2 - \hat{V}_z^2)^{1/2} \sqrt{\frac{M-m}{M-1}} = 166.09$$

$$95\% \; CI = 4518.3 \pm (1.96 * 166.09) = (4192.76, 4843.84)$$

$$x'' = x' * \frac{Z}{z'} = 30 * \frac{7217}{3530} = 61.3$$

$$\widehat{SE}(x'') = \frac{Z * r}{\sqrt{m}} (\hat{V}_x^2 + \hat{V}_z^2 - 2\hat{\rho}_{xz}\hat{V}_x\hat{V}_z)^{1/2} \sqrt{\frac{M-m}{M-1}}$$

$$\hat{\rho}_{xz} \approx \frac{\hat{V}_x}{\hat{V}_z}$$

$$\widehat{SE}(x'') = \frac{Z * r}{\sqrt{m}} (\hat{V}_x^2 - \hat{V}_z^2)^{1/2} \sqrt{\frac{M-m}{M-1}} = 14.22$$

$$95\% \; CI = 61.3 \pm (1.96 * 14.22) = (33.43, 89.17)$$

Using STATA, we get the following estimated totals, standard errors, and confidence intervals. The standard errors computed by STATA are different compared to the ones computed by hand. In the hand calculations an approximation of the correlation was used. This approximation does not always work well and hence we should be more confident using the standard error computed by STATA. The confidence intervals also differ because the standard errors differ and also because STATA uses the t-distribution instead of the standard normal distribution.

```
. gen M = 33

. gen wt = M / 10

. svyset _n [pweight=wt], fpc(M)

      pweight: wt
          VCE: linearized
  Single unit: missing
     Strata 1: <one>
         SU 1: <observations>
        FPC 1: M

. gen pat_infl= tot_pat*7217

. svy: ratio  pat_infl  num_beds
(running ratio on estimation sample)

Survey: Ratio estimation

Number of strata =          1        Number of obs     =        10
Number of PSUs   =         10        Population size   =        33
                                     Design df         =         9

    _ratio_1: pat_infl/num_beds

-----------------------------------------------------------------
             |               Linearized
             |      Ratio    Std. Err.     [95% Conf. Interval]
-------------+---------------------------------------------------
    _ratio_1 |   4518.292    172.4057      4128.283     4908.301
-----------------------------------------------------------------

. gen dead_infl= tot_dead*7217

. svy: ratio  dead_infl  num_beds
(running ratio on estimation sample)

Survey: Ratio estimation

Number of strata =          1        Number of obs     =        10
Number of PSUs   =         10        Population size   =        33
                                     Design df         =         9

    _ratio_1: dead_infl/num_beds

-----------------------------------------------------------------
             |               Linearized
             |      Ratio    Std. Err.     [95% Conf. Interval]
-------------+---------------------------------------------------
    _ratio_1 |   61.33428    14.76202      27.94026      94.7283
-----------------------------------------------------------------
```

9.5 *A survey which used a simple one-stage cluster sampling design was conducted in a large city in China. The clusters in this instance were entities known as "neighborhood groups" (translated from the Chinese "jumin xiaozu"), which are essentially groups of contiguous households. These so-called neighborhood groups are the smallest units for which population information is available in the Peoples Republic of China (PRC). The city comprises six districts which, in this design, comprise the strata. Within each district, a simple random sample of two neighborhood groups was selected, and all individuals within each neighborhood group were interviewed concerning their overall health status. The following represents data from the survey on the number of individuals over 30 years of age who were edentulous.*

District	Neighborhood Group	Number of Persons > 30 years	Number of Edentulous Persons
1	1	28	7
	2	35	9
2	1	29	12
	2	43	26
3	1	61	19
	2	48	12
4	1	15	10
	2	39	28
5	1	21	9
	2	46	15
6	1	12	0
	2	25	4

Strata 1, 2, 4, and 6 each contain 200 neighborhood groups; stratum 3 contains 175 neighborhood groups; and stratum 5 contains 150 neighborhood groups. Estimate and construct 95% confidence intervals for (1) the total number of edentulous persons 30 years of age and over, and (2) the proportion of all persons 30 years of age and older who are edentulous.

Solution: In this problem, the clusters are the neighborhood groups and the strata are the six districts. Let $m = 2$, $M_1 = M_2 = M_4 = M_6 = 200$, $M_3 = 175$, and $M_5 = 150$.

$$x'_{str,clu} = \sum_{h=1}^{L} \frac{M_h}{m_h} x_h = \frac{200}{2} * (16 + 38 + 38 + 4) + \frac{175}{2} * 31 + \frac{150}{2} * 24 = 14{,}112.5$$

Let $\hat{\sigma}^2_{1hx}$ be the variance among listing units in each stratum.

$$\widehat{Var}(x'_{str,clu}) = \sum_{h=1}^{L} \frac{M_h^2}{m_h} * \hat{\sigma}_{1hx}^2 * \left(\frac{M_h - m_h}{M_h - 1} \right)$$

$$= \frac{200^2}{2}(2 + 98 + 162 + 8) * \frac{198}{199} + \frac{175^2}{2}(24.5)\frac{173}{174} + \frac{150^2}{2} * 18 * \frac{148}{149}$$

$$= 5{,}947{,}005$$

$$\widehat{SE}(x'_{str,clu}) = 2438.6$$

$$95\% \ CI = 14112.5 \pm (1.96 * 2438.6) = (9333, 18{,}893)$$

Next, we will use Equations 7.18 and 7.19 to estimate the ratio and obtain a 95% confidence interval.

$$y'_{str,clu} = \sum_{h=1}^{L} \frac{M_h}{m_h} y_h = \frac{200}{2} * (63 + 72 + 54 + 37) + \frac{175}{2} * 109 + \frac{150}{2} * 67$$

$$= 37{,}162.5$$

$$r_{str,clu} = \frac{14{,}112.5}{37{,}162.5} = 0.3798$$

$$\widehat{Var}(r_{str,clu}) = \frac{1}{M^2 \bar{Y}^2} \sum_{h=1}^{L} \frac{M_h^2(M_h - m_h)}{m_h(M_h - 1)} \hat{\sigma}_{hz}^2$$

$$\hat{\sigma}_{hz}^2 = \hat{\sigma}_{hx}^2 + \hat{r}_{str,clu}^2 \hat{\sigma}_{hy}^2 - 2\hat{r}_{str,clu}^2 \hat{\rho}_{hxy} \hat{\sigma}_{hx} \hat{\sigma}_{hy}$$

We cannot calculate $\hat{\rho}_{hxy}$ separately for each stratum because we only have 2 clusters within each one, thus $\hat{\rho}_{hxy} = 1$. We can calculate $\hat{\rho}_{hxy}$ over all strata and assume that the overall coefficient is the same for each stratum. This estimate is $\hat{\rho}_{hxy} = 0.66$.

116 CHAPTER 9 SOLUTIONS

$$\widehat{Var}(r_{str,clu}) = \frac{1}{M^2\bar{Y}^2} \sum_{h=1}^{L} \frac{M_h^2(M_h - m_h)}{m_h(M_h - 1)} \hat{\sigma}_{hz}^2$$

$$= \frac{1}{1125^2 * 33.5^2}$$

$$* \left[\frac{200^2 * 198}{2(199)} (2.025 + 63.005 + 95.255 + 7.154) + \frac{175^2 * 173}{2(174)} (13.878) \right.$$

$$\left. + \frac{150^2 * 148}{2(149)} (25.477) \right] = 0.0027$$

$$95\% \ CI = 0.3798 \pm \left(1.96 * 0.0027^{1/2} \right) = (0.278, 0.4816)$$

Using STATA, we get the estimates below. Recall, the standard errors and confidence intervals will differ slightly between the hand calculations and STATA due to the fact that STATA uses different procedures in their construction.

```
. gen wt=200/2

. replace wt = 175 / 2 if district == 3
(2 real changes made)

. replace wt = 150 / 2 if district == 5
(2 real changes made)

. svyset  nbhd_grp [pweight= wt], strata( district)

      pweight: wt
          VCE: linearized
  Single unit: missing
     Strata 1: district
         SU 1: nbhd_grp
        FPC 1: <zero>

. svy: total   num_ednt
(running total on estimation sample)

Survey: Total estimation

Number of strata =        6      Number of obs    =       12
Number of PSUs   =       12      Population size  =     1125
                                 Design df        =        6

-------------------------------------------------------------
             |             Linearized
             |    Total    Std. Err.    [95% Conf. Interval]
-------------+-----------------------------------------------
   num_ednt  |   14112.5   2444.925     8129.985    20095.01
-------------------------------------------------------------




. svy: total   num_30
(running total on estimation sample)
```

```
Survey: Total estimation

Number of strata   =        6        Number of obs     =       12
Number of PSUs     =       12        Population size   =     1125
                                     Design df         =        6

-----------------------------------------------------------------
                  |              Linearized
                  |     Total    Std. Err.    [95% Conf. Interval]
------------------+----------------------------------------------
          num_30  |   37162.5    3835.301     27777.86    46547.14
-----------------------------------------------------------------
```

For the proportion of edentulous persons we get from STATA:

```
. svy: ratio  num_ednt num_30
(running ratio on estimation sample)

Survey: Ratio estimation

Number of strata =        6        Number of obs     =       12
Number of PSUs   =       12        Population size   =     1125
                                   Design df         =        6

    _ratio_1: num_ednt/num_30

-----------------------------------------------------------------
                  |              Linearized
                  |     Ratio    Std. Err.    [95% Conf. Interval]
------------------+----------------------------------------------
        _ratio_1  |  .3797511    .0346487     .2949688    .4645334
-----------------------------------------------------------------
```

9.6 *In Exercise 9.5, it was discovered during the field work that sample neighborhood group 2 in District 3 no longer existed because of redistribution of the population. With this in mind, obtain modified estimates of the parameters estimated in Exercise 9.5.*

Solution: In this problem, the clusters are the neighborhood groups and the strata are the six districts. Let $m = 2$ for strata 1, 2, 4, 5, and 6; and $m = 1$ for stratum 3. Let $M_1 = M_2 = M_4 = M_6 = 200$, $M_3 = 174$, and $M_5 = 150$.

$$x'_{str,clu} = \sum_{h=1}^{L} \frac{M_h}{m_h} x_h = \frac{200}{2} * (16 + 38 + 38 + 4) + \frac{174}{1} * 19 + \frac{150}{2} * 24 = 14,706$$

Let $\hat{\sigma}^2_{1hx}$ be the variance among listing units in each stratum.

$$\widehat{Var}(x'_{str,clu}) = \sum_{h=1}^{L} \frac{M_h^2}{m_h} * \hat{\sigma}^2_{1hx} * \left(\frac{M_h - m_h}{M_h - 1}\right)$$

$$= \frac{200^2}{2}(2 + 98 + 162 + 8) * \frac{198}{199} + \frac{174^2}{1}(0)\frac{172}{173} + \frac{150^2}{2} * 18 * \frac{148}{149}$$

$$= 5,574,005$$

$$\widehat{SE}(x'_{str,clu}) = 2360.9$$

$$95\% \ CI = 14706 \pm (1.96 * 2360.9) = (10,079, 19,333)$$

Next, we will use Equations 7.18 and 7.19 to estimate the ratio and obtain a 95% confidence interval.

$$y'_{str,clu} = \sum_{h=1}^{L} \frac{M_h}{m_h} y_h = \frac{200}{2} * (63 + 72 + 54 + 37) + \frac{174}{1} * 61 + \frac{150}{2} * 67 = 38,239$$

$$r_{str,clu} = \frac{14,706}{38,239} = 0.3846$$

$$\widehat{Var}(r_{str,clu}) = \frac{1}{M^2 \bar{Y}^2} \sum_{h=1}^{L} \frac{M_h^2(M_h - m_h)}{m_h(M_h - 1)} \hat{\sigma}^2_{hz}$$

$$\hat{\sigma}^2_{hz} = \hat{\sigma}^2_{hx} + \hat{r}^2_{str,clu}\hat{\sigma}^2_{hy} - 2\hat{r}^2_{str,clu}\hat{\rho}_{hxy}\hat{\sigma}_{hx}\hat{\sigma}_{hy}$$

We cannot calculate $\hat{\rho}_{hxy}$ separately for each stratum because we only have 2 clusters within each one, thus $\hat{\rho}_{hxy} = 1$. We can calculate $\hat{\rho}_{hxy}$ over all strata and assume that the overall coefficient is the same for each stratum. This estimate is $\hat{\rho}_{hxy} = 0.699$.

$$\widehat{Var}(r_{str,clu}) = \frac{1}{M^2\bar{Y}^2} \sum_{h=1}^{L} \frac{M_h^2(M_h - m_h)}{m_h(M_h - 1)} \hat{\sigma}_{hz}^2$$

$$= \frac{1}{1125^2 * 32.2^2}$$

$$* \left[\frac{200^2 * 198}{2(199)} (2.025 + 63.005 + 95.255 + 7.154) + \frac{174^2 * 173}{2(173)} (0) \right.$$

$$\left. + \frac{150^2 * 148}{2(149)} (25.477) \right] = 0.0026$$

$$95\% \ CI = 0.3846 \pm \left(1.96 * 0.0026^{1/2} \right) = (0.2847, 0.4845$$

9.7   *A dental HMO has 368 members and each member has 4 quadrants (upper left, upper right, lower left, lower right). It is desired to conduct a sample survey with the objective in mind of estimating the total number of quadrants among the membership that require some form of periodontal surgery. The sampling plan would involve taking a simple random sample of patients and evaluating, for each sample patient, the status of each of the four quadrants. A preliminary study, based on a judgmental sample of 7 patients, yielded the following data:*

	Quadrant			
Patient	*1*	*2*	*3*	*4*
1	+	+	+	--
2	--	--	+	+
3	--	--	--	--
4	+	--	--	+
5	--	--	--	--
6	+	--	--	--
7	+	+	+	+

where 1 = lower left, 2 = lower right, 3 = upper left, 4 = upper right, + = requires surgery, -- = does not require surgery.

Based on these preliminary data, how many patients are required if it is desired to estimate, with 95% certainty, the total number of quadrants among all members that require periodontal surgery to within 15% of the true value?

Solution: We will take a simple random sample of patients, where each patient is a cluster. Let $M = 368$ and $m = 7$, $z = 1.96$ and $\varepsilon = 0.15$.

We will use the sample size equation in Box 9.4 to calculate this sample size.

$$m = \frac{z_{1-\alpha/_2}^2 * M * \hat{V}_{1x}^2}{z_{1-\alpha/_2}^2 * \hat{V}_{1x}^2 + (M-1) * \varepsilon^2}$$

$$\hat{V}_{1x}^2 = \frac{\hat{\sigma}_{1x}^2}{\bar{x}^2} = \frac{\frac{367}{368} * 2.238}{1.714^2} = 0.759$$

$$m = \frac{1.96^2 * 368 * 0.759}{1.96^2 * 0.759 + 359 * 0.15^2} = \frac{1073}{11.17} = 96.03 \text{ or } 97$$

9.8   *In the scenario described in Exercise 9.7, it is anticipated that it would take about 15 min for a dentist to examine each quadrant, and that it would take approximately 20 min of clerical time to schedule the appointment for each patient sampled and to prepare the patient for the examination. If these are the only costs involved in the survey, and if clerical time is one-third as expensive as dentist's time, what budget (expressed in dentist person-hours) would be required to meet the specifications stated in Exercise 9.7?*

Solution: Both the dentist time and clerical time will be expressed in dentist hours. The clerical time is equal to $C_{clerical} = (1/3 \text{ hour} * 1/3) * 97 = 10.78$ hours. The dentist time is equal to $C_{dentist} = (1/4 \text{ hour}) * 97 * 4 = 97$. Thus, the total time in dentist hours is equal to 107.78 hours.

9.9   *In many health science situations, a cluster consists of a pair of elements (e.g., in ophthalmology, clusters might be patients; elements might be eyes, etc.). In this situation, derive a simplified expression for the variance of an estimated total.*

Solution:

$$\widehat{SE}(x'_{clu}) = \frac{M}{\sqrt{m}}\hat{\sigma}_{1x}\sqrt{\frac{M-m}{M-1}}$$

$$\hat{\sigma}_{1x} = \left[\frac{\sum_{i=1}^{m}(x_i - \bar{x}_{clu})^2}{m-1}\right]^{1/2}\sqrt{\frac{M-1}{M}}$$

But, for a cluster of size 2,

$$\left[\frac{\sum_{i=1}^{m}(x_i - \bar{x}_{clu})^2}{(m-1)}\right]^{1/2} = \left[\frac{\sum_{i=1}^{m}(x_{i1} - x_{i2})^2}{2*(m-1)}\right]^{1/2}$$

Therefore,

$$\widehat{SE}(x'_{clu})$$

$$= \frac{M}{\sqrt{m}}\left[\frac{\sum_{i=1}^{m}(x_{i1} - x_{i2})^2}{2*(m-1)}\right]^{1/2}\sqrt{\frac{M-1}{M}}\sqrt{\frac{M-m}{M-1}} = \frac{M}{\sqrt{m}}\left[\frac{\sum_{i=1}^{m}(x_{i1} - x_{i2})^2}{2*(m-1)}\right]^{1/2}\sqrt{M-m}$$

9.10   *In the situation described in Exercise 9.9, derive a simplified expression for the variance of an estimated ratio.*

Solution:

$$\widehat{SE}(r_{clu}) = r_{clu}$$

$$* \left\{ \frac{\left[\widehat{SE}(\bar{x}_{clu})\right]^2}{\bar{x}_{clu}^2} + \frac{\left[\widehat{SE}(\bar{y}_{clu})\right]^2}{\bar{y}_{clu}^2} - \frac{2}{m} * \left(\frac{M-m}{M}\right) * \left(\frac{1}{\bar{x}_{clu}\bar{y}_{clu}}\right) \right.$$

$$\left. * \frac{\sum_{i=1}^{m}(x_i - \bar{x}_{clu})(y_i - \bar{y}_{clu})}{m-1} \right\}^{1/2}$$

$$= r_{clu}$$

$$* \left\{ \frac{\left[\frac{1}{m} * \left[\frac{\sum_{i=1}^{m}(x_{i1} - x_{i2})^2}{2*(m-1)}\right]^{1/2} * \sqrt{\frac{M-m}{M}}\right]^2}{\bar{x}_{clu}^2} \right.$$

$$+ \frac{\left[\frac{1}{m} * \left[\frac{\sum_{i=1}^{m}(y_{i1} - y_{i2})^2}{2*(m-1)}\right]^{1/2} * \sqrt{\frac{M-m}{M}}\right]^2}{\bar{y}_{clu}^2} - \frac{2}{m} * \left(\frac{M-m}{M}\right) * \left(\frac{1}{\bar{x}_{clu}\bar{y}_{clu}}\right)$$

$$\left. * \frac{\sum_{i=1}^{m}(x_i - \bar{x}_{clu})(y_i - \bar{y}_{clu})}{2*(m-1)} \right\}^{1/2}$$

9.11   *Suppose that 40,000 person-hours were allotted for field costs for the sample survey of district courts discussed in an illustrative example in this chapter. Using the cost functions and cost components developed for this example, determine which of the two sample designs—simple one-stage cluster sampling or simple random sampling—would estimate the total number of persons receiving treatment for substance abuse with the lower standard error.*

Solution: For the simple random sample with 40,000 person-hours allotted for field costs, we have:

$$n = \frac{C - C_0}{C_1} = \frac{40,000 - 34,142}{0.75} \approx 7811$$

The standard error of the total can be found using the following formula:

$$SE(x') = \frac{N\sqrt{P(1 - P)}}{\sqrt{n}} * \sqrt{\frac{N - n}{N - 1}}$$

Let $N = 15,364$, $n = 7811$, and $P = 2444 / 15364 = 0.159$

$$SE(x') = \frac{15,364\sqrt{0.159(1 - 0.159)}}{\sqrt{7811}} * \sqrt{\frac{15,364 - 7811}{15363 - 1}} = 44.58$$

If we assume 40,000 for the one-stage cluster design, then:

$$40,000 = 1313.17 * m + 0.75 * m * 590.9 = m(1313.17 + 443.2) = 1756.4m$$

$$m \approx 23$$

Assuming 23 clusters are sampled, and holding the specifications in the book example equal, the standard error associated with cluster sampling is:

$$\widehat{SE}(x'_{clu}) = \frac{M}{\sqrt{m}}\hat{\sigma}_{1x}\sqrt{\frac{M - m}{M - 1}} = \frac{26}{\sqrt{23}}128.86\sqrt{\frac{3}{25}} = 242.0$$

The standard error associated with the one-stage cluster sample is still larger than the simple random sampling estimated standard error.

9.12   For the sample survey of district courts discussed in an illustrative example in this chapter, draw a graph with the abscissa being total fixed costs and the ordinate being the coefficient of variation of the estimated total number of persons receiving treatment for substance abuse. The graph should have two lines (similar to Figure 9.2): one for a simple one-stage sample design; the other for a simple random sampling design.

Solution: In this problem, we will follow the procedure that was used for Exercise 9.11. That is, for a given cost we will estimate the coefficient of variation for simple one-stage cluster sampling and the coefficient of variation for simple random sampling. The range on the x-axis is 35,000 person hours to 43,000 because you need at least 34,142 person hours to construct the frame for simple random sampling, hence the lower bound. For cluster sampling, if the costs are 44,000 then the standard error is zero (and above 44,000 the standard error is negative).

We see in the plot that simple random sampling results in a lower coefficient of variation compared to one-stage cluster sampling at all costs considered.

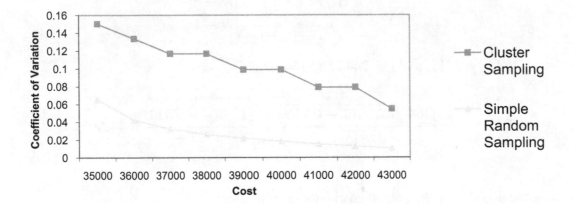

Chapter Ten – Solutions

10.1 *Suppose that Chicago is divided into 75 community areas and that each community area contains 20 retail pharmacies. Suppose that you wish to estimate the average prices charged for some standard prescription drugs by taking a simple random sample of eight community areas followed by a simple random sample of four pharmacies within each of the eight community areas selected.*

a. *Prepare a simple cost function for estimating the overall survey cost including the field costs. Specify each of the cost components.*

Solution: In a two-stage cluster design, the cost function can be approximated by Equation 10.8:

$$C = C_1^* m + C_1^* m \bar{n}$$

The first component includes the costs associated with traveling to each sample cluster for the purpose of listing the sampling units, the cost of listing the listing units, the cost of selecting the sample from each list, and the cost of traveling back to the cluster to do the interviewing. The second component covers the cost of interviewing each of the sampling units selected.

In this problem, $M = 75, m = 8, \bar{N} = 20$ and $\bar{n} = 4$.

We can assume that the cost associated with traveling to the clusters, listing the units, selecting the sample, and traveling back for interviewing is $100 per cluster (approximately 5 hours at $20 per hour). The cost of interviewing each of the sampled units selected can be set to $40 (approximately 2 hours at $20 per hour).

Thus, the total cost is $C = 100(8) + 40(8)(4) = 800 + 1280$
   $= \$2080.$

b. *How would the total cost indicated above be affected if 16 community areas and two pharmacies per community area were selected?*

Solution: The new specifications would change the total cost the following way:

$$C = 100(16) + 40(16)(2) = 1600 + 1280 = \$2880.$$

This sampling plan would cost an additional $800 to complete. It would be more economical to travel to fewer areas and perform more interviews within each sampled area.

c.   *Suppose it is guessed that the standard deviation σ_x among all stores in Chicago with respect to the price of a certain drug is \$4.50 and that the average cost of this drug is \$30.00. Using the cost function you specified in part (a), determine the optimum value of $\bar{n}$ if the intraclass correlation coefficient is equal to 0.35. What then would be the coefficient of variation of the estimate if six PSUs were used?*

Solution:

$$We\ will\ use\ Equation\ 10.9\ to\ estimate\ the\ value\ of\ \bar{n}.$$

$$\bar{n} = \left[\left(\frac{C_1^*}{C_2^*} \right) \left(\frac{1 - \delta_x}{\delta_x} \right) \right]^{1/2} = \left[\left(\frac{100}{40} \right) \left(\frac{1 - 0.35}{0.35} \right) \right]^{1/2} = 2.15 = 3$$

Equation 10.15 will be used to estimate the standard error, and then the standard equation will be used to estimate the coefficient of variation.

$$\widehat{SE}(\bar{\bar{x}}_{clu}) = \left(\frac{\sigma_x}{\sqrt{n}} \right) \sqrt{1 + \delta_x(\bar{n} - 1)} = \left(\frac{4.5}{\sqrt{18}} \right) \sqrt{1 + 0.35(3 - 1)} = 1.383$$

$$\widehat{V}(\bar{\bar{x}}_{clu}) = \frac{1.383}{30} = 0.0461$$

10.2 *a. Suppose that the elementary schools in a city were grouped into 30 school districts, with each school district containing ten schools. Suppose that a simple random sample of three school districts was taken and that within each sample school district a simple random sample of four schools was taken for purposes of estimating the number of school children in the city that are color-blind (as measured by a standard test). The data shown in the accompanying table were obtained from this sample. Estimate, and obtain a 95% confidence interval for, the total number of color-blind school children in the city.*

Sample School District	Sample School	Number of Children	Number of Color-Blind Children
1	1	130	2
	2	150	3
	3	160	3
	4	120	5
2	1	110	2
	2	120	4
	3	100	0
	4	120	1
3	1	89	4
	2	130	2
	3	100	0
	4	150	2

Solution: First, enter the data into STATA's data editor.

```
. list

      district    school   tot_chld   cbl_chld
 1.       1          1        130          2
 2.       1          2        150          3
 3.       1          3        160          3
 4.       1          4        120          5
 5.       2          1        110          2
 6.       2          2        120          4
 7.       2          3        100          0
 8.       2          4        120          1
 9.       3          1         89          4
10.       3          2        130          2
11.       3          3        100          0
12.       3          4        150          2
```

Next, use the following commands to estimate the total and 95% confidence interval.

```
. gen wt = 1 / ((3/30)*(4/10))

. svyset district [pweight=wt]
       pweight: wt
           VCE: linearized
  Single unit: missing
     Strata 1: <one>
         SU 1: district
        FPC 1: <zero>

. svy: total cbl_chld
(running total on estimation sample)

Survey: Total estimation

Number of strata =        1        Number of obs    =      12
Number of PSUs   =        3        Population size  =     300
                                   Design df        =       2


------------------------------------------------------------
              |              Linearized
              |     Total   Std. Err.    [95% Conf. Interval]
--------------+---------------------------------------------
     cbl_chld |       700   139.1941     101.0961    1298.904
------------------------------------------------------------
```

The estimated total number of color-blind children in the city is 700 and the 95% confidence interval for this estimate is 101.1 to 1298.9.

b.   *Estimate, and obtain a 95% confidence interval for, the proportion of school children in the city who are color-blind.*

Solution: We will use the svy: ratio procedure in STATA to obtain this estimate and 95% confidence interval.

```
. svy: ratio  cbl_chld tot_chld
(running ratio on estimation sample)

Survey: Ratio estimation

Number of strata =        1        Number of obs    =      12
Number of PSUs   =        3        Population size  =     300
                                   Design df        =       2

     _ratio_1: cbl_chld/tot_chld


------------------------------------------------------------
              |              Linearized
              |     Ratio   Std. Err.    [95% Conf. Interval]
--------------+---------------------------------------------
     _ratio_1 | .0189317    .002461      .0083428    .0295206
------------------------------------------------------------
```

The estimated proportion of color-blind children in the city is 0.019 and the 95% confidence interval for this estimate is 0.008 to 0.030.

10.3 *A simple random sample requires 400 listing units in order for estimated means and totals to meet specifications of precision. If all PSUs have the same number $\overline{N}$ of listing units, how large a simple cluster sample with cluster size $\overline{n}$ equal to 4 would be needed to achieve the same precision when the intraclass correlation coefficient is equal to 0.6?*

Solution: To solve this problem, set the standard error of the mean under simple random sampling equal to the standard error of the mean under cluster sampling.

$$\widehat{SE}(\bar{\bar{x}}_{srs}) = \frac{\sigma_x}{\sqrt{n}}$$

$$\widehat{SE}(\bar{\bar{x}}_{clu}) = \frac{\sigma_x}{\sqrt{m\bar{n}}}\sqrt{1 + \delta_x(\bar{n} - 1)}$$

$$\frac{\sigma_x}{\sqrt{400}} = \left(\frac{\sigma_x}{\sqrt{4m}}\right)\sqrt{1 + 0.60(4 - 1)}$$

$$\frac{2\sqrt{m}}{\sqrt{400}} = 1.6733$$

$$m = 280$$

10.4 *Suppose that during the peak season the number of visitors to a state park and the number of injuries occurring among these visitors are as given in the accompanying table by week and day (the park is closed on Fridays).*

| Week | \multicolumn{6}{c|}{Number of Visitors} | \multicolumn{6}{c|}{Number of Injuries} |
	Su	M	Tu	W	Th	Sa	Su	M	Tu	W	Th	Sa
1	200	150	130	140	150	190	2	3	1	4	3	8
2	120	105	111	103	111	130	1	0	0	1	0	3
3	310	200	180	130	125	208	4	0	1	0	1	3
4	200	107	101	98	103	137	3	0	2	0	1	8
5	170	160	130	121	107	114	3	0	0	1	0	5
6	250	237	209	212	231	180	2	0	0	0	0	1
7	380	378	325	330	306	331	4	3	0	8	0	2
8	495	400	315	302	350	395	4	0	3	2	2	4
9	206	200	108	95	107	190	1	2	3	0	1	4
10	308	300	293	206	200	300	0	0	1	2	0	3

Suppose that a simple two-stage cluster sample was taken with weeks as clusters, days as listing units, m = 4 and $\overline{n}$ = 3. Suppose further that at the first stage of sampling, clusters 2, 6, 8, and 10 are selected. At the second stage of sampling, let us suppose that listing units 2, 3, and 5 are selected within cluster 2; listing units 1, 3, and 6 are selected within cluster 6; listing units 3, 4, and 6 are selected within cluster 8; and listing units 2, 4, and 5 are selected within cluster 10. From this sample, estimate and give 95% confidence intervals for the following:

a.   *The total number of visitors during the peak season.*

Solution: We will use STATA to complete this problem. First, enter the data into STATA's data editor.

```
.  list

        Week        Day   Visitors   Injuries
  1.       2          2        105          0
  2.       2          3        111          0
  3.       2          5        111          0
  4.       6          1        250          2
  5.       6          3        209          0
  6.       6          6        180          1
  7.       8          3        315          3
  8.       8          4        302          2
  9.       8          6        395          4
 10.      10          2        300          0
 11.      10          4        206          2
 12.      10          5        200          0
```

Next, we will use the svy: total procedure to obtain the estimated total number of visitors and a 95% confidence interval for that estimate.

The sampling weight is the inverse of the overall sampling fraction.

```
. gen wt = 1 / ((4/10)*(3/6))

. gen N=60

. gen M=10

. svyset week [pweight=wt], fpc(M) || _n, fpc(N)
      pweight: wt
          VCE: linearized
  Single unit: missing
     Strata 1: <one>
         SU 1: week
        FPC 1: M
     Strata 2: <one>
         SU 2: <observations>
        FPC 2: N

. svy: total visitors
(running total on estimation sample)

Survey: Total estimation

Number of strata =          1      Number of obs    =       12
Number of PSUs   =          4      Population size  =       60
                                   Design df        =        3


-----------------------------------------------------------------
              |              Linearized
              |     Total   Std. Err.    [95% Conf. Interval]
--------------+--------------------------------------------------
     visitors |     13420   2221.451      6350.352    20489.65
-----------------------------------------------------------------
```

The estimated total number of visitors is 13,420. A 95% confidence interval for that estimate is 6350 to 20490.

Note, the estimated total and standard error for this estimate can be calculated using the equations in Box 10.2.

$$y'_{clu} = \frac{x}{y} = \frac{2684}{1/5} = 13,420$$

$$\widehat{SE}(y'_{clu}) = \left(\frac{M}{\sqrt{m}f_2}\right)\left[\frac{\sum_{i=1}^{m}(y_i - \bar{y})^2}{m-1}\right]^{1/2}\left(\frac{N-n}{N}\right)^{1/2}$$

$$\frac{\sum_{i=1}^{m}(y_i - \bar{y})^2}{m-1}$$
$$= \frac{(327 - 671)^2 + (639 - 671)^2 + (1012 - 671)^2 + (706 - 671)^2}{3}$$
$$= 78,955.3$$

$$\widehat{SE}(y'_{clu}) = \left(\frac{10}{\sqrt{4}(3/6)}\right)[78,955.3]^{1/2}\left(\frac{60-12}{60}\right)^{1/2} = 2513.25$$

Notice, the estimated standard error is different from the one that is computed using STATA. The reason is that STATA uses a different procedure from the one in Box 10.2 for calculating the standard error under a two-stage cluster sampling plan.

b.   *The total number of injuries during the peak season.*

Solution: Again, we will use the svy: total procedure in STATA.

```
. svy: total  injuries
(running total on estimation sample)

Survey: Total estimation

Number of strata =        1         Number of obs    =       12
Number of PSUs   =        4         Population size  =       60
                                    Design df        =        3


-------------------------------------------------------------------
             |               Linearized
             |      Total     Std. Err.      [95% Conf. Interval]
-------------+-----------------------------------------------------
   injuries  |         70     31.54362       -30.38588    170.3859
-------------------------------------------------------------------
```

The estimated total number of injuries is 70 and the 95% confidence interval for this estimate is 0 to 170.

Again, we can compute this estimate and standard error using the equations in Box 10.2. As before, the standard error estimate calculated using the equation in Box 10.2 is different from the estimate computed in STATA.

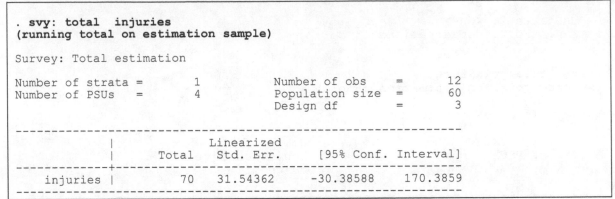

$$y'_{clu} = \frac{x}{y} = \frac{14}{1/5} = 70$$

$$\widehat{SE}(x'_{clu}) = \left(\frac{M}{\sqrt{m}f_2}\right)\left[\frac{\sum_{i=1}^{m}(x_i - \bar{x})^2}{m-1}\right]^{1/2}\left(\frac{N-n}{N}\right)^{1/2}$$

$$\frac{\sum_{i=1}^{m}(x_i - \bar{x})^2}{m-1} = \frac{(0 - 3.5)^2 + (3 - 3.5)^2 + (9 - 3.5)^2 + (2 - 3.5)^2}{3} = 15$$

$$\widehat{SE}(x'_{clu}) = \left(\frac{10}{\sqrt{4}(3/6)}\right)[15]^{1/2}\left(\frac{60-12}{60}\right)^{1/2} = 34.64$$

c. *The total number of injuries and visitors per week.*

Solution:

```
. gen vis_wk = Visitors / 10

. gen inj_wk = Injuries / 10

. svy: total  vis_wk
(running total on estimation sample)

Survey: Total estimation

Number of strata =        1            Number of obs    =      12
Number of PSUs   =        4            Population size  =      60
                                       Design df        =       3

----------------------------------------------------------------
              |                Linearized
              |     Total    Std. Err.      [95% Conf. Interval]
--------------+-------------------------------------------------
       vis_wk |      1342    222.1451       635.0352    2048.965
----------------------------------------------------------------

. svy: total inj_wk
(running total on estimation sample)

Survey: Total estimation

Number of strata =        1            Number of obs    =      12
Number of PSUs   =        4            Population size  =      60
                                       Design df        =       3

----------------------------------------------------------------
              |                Linearized
              |     Total    Std. Err.      [95% Conf. Interval]
--------------+-------------------------------------------------
       inj_wk |         7    3.154362      -3.038588    17.03859
----------------------------------------------------------------
```

The total number of visitors per week is estimated to be 1342 and the 95% confidence interval for this estimate is 635 to 2049. The total number of injuries per week is estimated to be 7 and the 95% confidence interval is 0 to 17.

The estimated totals and standard errors can be calculated using the equations in Box 10.2. The standard errors are slightly different from the ones obtained using STATA.

$$\bar{y}_{clu} = \frac{y'_{clu}}{m} = \frac{13420}{10} = 1342$$

$$\widehat{SE}(\bar{y}_{clu}) = \left(\frac{\widehat{SE}(y'_{clu})}{10}\right) = 251.33$$

$$\bar{x}_{clu} = \frac{x'_{clu}}{m} = \frac{70}{10} = 7$$

$$\widehat{SE}(\bar{x}_{clu}) = \left(\frac{\widehat{SE}(x'_{clu})}{10}\right) = 3.46$$

d.   *The total number of injuries and visitors per day.*

Solution:

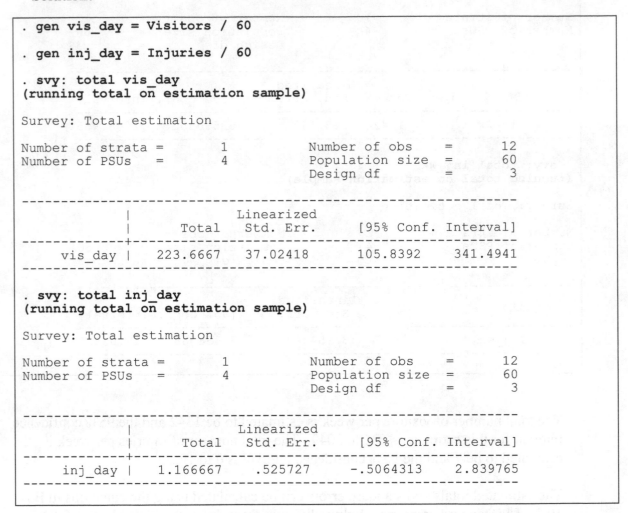

```
. gen vis_day = Visitors / 60

. gen inj_day = Injuries / 60

. svy: total vis_day
(running total on estimation sample)

Survey: Total estimation

Number of strata =        1          Number of obs    =       12
Number of PSUs   =        4          Population size  =       60
                                     Design df        =        3

------------------------------------------------------------------
               |               Linearized
               |      Total   Std. Err.      [95% Conf. Interval]
---------------+--------------------------------------------------
      vis_day  |   223.6667   37.02418       105.8392    341.4941
------------------------------------------------------------------

. svy: total inj_day
(running total on estimation sample)

Survey: Total estimation

Number of strata =        1          Number of obs    =       12
Number of PSUs   =        4          Population size  =       60
                                     Design df        =        3

------------------------------------------------------------------
               |               Linearized
               |      Total   Std. Err.      [95% Conf. Interval]
---------------+--------------------------------------------------
      inj_day  |   1.166667    .525727      -.5064313    2.839765
------------------------------------------------------------------
```

The estimated number of visitors per day is 224 and the 95% confidence interval is 106 to 341. The estimated number of injuries per day is 1.2 and the 95% confidence interval for this estimate is 0 to 3.

The equations in Box 10.2 will be used next to compute these estimates and standard errors.

$$\bar{\bar{y}}_{clu} = \frac{y'_{clu}}{N} = \frac{13420}{60} = 223.667$$

$$\widehat{SE}(\bar{\bar{y}}_{clu}) = \left(\frac{\widehat{SE}(\bar{y}_{clu})}{6}\right) = 41.89$$

$$\bar{\bar{x}}_{clu} = \frac{x'_{clu}}{m} = \frac{70}{60} = 1.167$$

$$\widehat{SE}(\bar{\bar{x}}_{clu}) = \left(\frac{\widehat{SE}(\bar{x}_{clu})}{6}\right) = 0.577$$

e.   *The number of injuries per visitor.*

Solution:

```
. svy: ratio  injuries visitors
(running ratio on estimation sample)

Survey: Ratio estimation

Number of strata =        1         Number of obs   =       12
Number of PSUs   =        4         Population size =       60
                                    Design df       =        3

    _ratio_1: injuries/visitors

---------------------------------------------------------------
             |              Linearized
             |      Ratio   Std. Err.    [95% Conf. Interval]
-------------+-------------------------------------------------
    _ratio_1 |   .0052161   .0016379    3.48e-06    .0104287
---------------------------------------------------------------
```

The estimated number of injuries per person is 0.005 and the 95% confidence interval is 0 to 0.010.

The equations for an estimated ratio and the standard error for this estimate are contained in Box 10.2. Note, the estimated standard error is different from the one computed by STATA.

$$r_{clu} = \frac{x}{y} = \frac{14}{2684} = 0.005$$

$$\widehat{SE}(r_{clu})$$

$$= r_{clu}\sqrt{\frac{N-n}{Nm}\left(\frac{\sum_{i=1}^{m}(x_i-\bar{x})^2}{(m-1)\bar{x}^2}+\frac{\sum_{i=1}^{m}(y_i-\bar{y})^2}{(m-1)\bar{y}^2}\right.}$$

$$\left.-2\frac{\sum_{i=1}^{m}(x_i-\bar{x})^2(y_i-\bar{y})^2}{(m-1)\bar{x}^2\bar{y}^2}\right)^{1/2}$$

$$= 0.005\sqrt{\frac{60-12}{60*4}\left(\frac{3.46^2}{7^2}+\frac{251.33^2}{1342^2}-2\frac{1014.33}{7*1342}\right)^{1/2}}$$

$$= 0.005*0.447*(0.244+0.035-0.216)^{1/2}=0.00056$$

10.5   *Suppose that a simple one-stage cluster sample was selected from the population shown in Exercise 10.4 and that clusters two and eight were selected. From this sample compute the 95% confidence interval for the characteristics given in parts (a)-(e) of Exercise 10.4.*

a.   *The total number of visitors during the peak season.*

Solution: First, enter the data into STATA's data editor.

```
. list

         Week      Day  Visitors  Injuries
  1.        2        1       120         1
  2.        2        2       105         0
  3.        2        3       111         0
  4.        2        4       103         1
  5.        2        5       111         0
  6.        2        6       130         3
  7.        8        1       495         4
  8.        8        2       400         0
  9.        8        3       315         3
 10.        8        4       302         2
 11.        8        5       350         2
 12.        8        6       395         4
```

Next, use the survey procedures in STATA to obtain the estimates and 95% confidence intervals.

```
. gen wt = 10 / 2

. gen M = 10

. svyset week [pweight=wt], fpc(M)

      pweight: wt
          VCE: linearized
  Single unit: missing
     Strata 1: <one>
         SU 1: week
        FPC 1: M

. svy: total visitors
(running total on estimation sample)

Survey: Total estimation

Number of strata =        1        Number of obs    =       12
Number of PSUs   =        2        Population size  =       60
                                   Design df        =        1


------------------------------------------------------------------
                 |              Linearized
                 |    Total    Std. Err.      [95% Conf. Interval]
-----------------+------------------------------------------------
      visitors   |    14685    7052.558      -74926.25    104296.3
------------------------------------------------------------------
```

The estimated total number of visitors is 14,685 and the 95% confidence interval is 0 to 104,296.

Note, a finite population correction was included in the survey procedure in STATA. This allowed us to obtain an estimated standard error that equals the standard error computed using the equations in Box 9.2.

b.   *The total number of injuries during the peak season.*

Solution:

```
. svy: total injuries
(running total on estimation sample)

Survey: Total estimation

Number of strata =        1        Number of obs    =       12
Number of PSUs   =        2        Population size  =       60
                                   Design df        =        1

--------------------------------------------------------------
             |              Linearized
             |    Total    Std. Err.    [95% Conf. Interval]
-------------+------------------------------------------------
    injuries |     100    44.72136    -468.2388     668.2388
--------------------------------------------------------------
```

The estimated total number of injuries is 100 and the 95% confidence interval is 0 to 668.

c.   *The total number of injuries and visitors per week.*

Solution:

```
. gen vis_wk = Visitors / 10

. gen inj_wk = Injuries / 10

. svy: total vis_wk
(running total on estimation sample)

Survey: Total estimation

Number of strata =        1        Number of obs    =       12
Number of PSUs   =        2        Population size  =       60
                                   Design df        =        1

--------------------------------------------------------------
             |              Linearized
             |    Total    Std. Err.    [95% Conf. Interval]
-------------+------------------------------------------------
      vis_wk |   1468.5   705.2558    -7492.625     10429.63
--------------------------------------------------------------
```

```
. svy: total inj_wk
(running total on estimation sample)
```

```
Survey: Total estimation

Number of strata =        1        Number of obs    =      12
Number of PSUs    =       2        Population size  =      60
                                   Design df        =       1

-----------------------------------------------------------
                 |            Linearized
                 |    Total   Std. Err.    [95% Conf. Interval]
-----------------+-----------------------------------------
          inj_wk |      10    4.472136    -46.82388    66.82388
-----------------------------------------------------------
```

The estimated number of visitors per week is 1469 and the 95% confidence interval is 0 to 10,430. The estimated number of injuries per week is 10 and the 95% confidence interval is 0 to 67.

d.   *The total number of injuries and visitors per day.*

Solution:

```
. gen vis_day = Visitors / 60

. gen inj_day = Injuries / 60


. svy: total vis_day
(running total on estimation sample)

Survey: Total estimation

Number of strata =        1        Number of obs    =      12
Number of PSUs    =       2        Population size  =      60
                                   Design df        =       1

-----------------------------------------------------------
                 |            Linearized
                 |    Total   Std. Err.    [95% Conf. Interval]
-----------------+-----------------------------------------
         vis_day |  244.75    117.5426    -1248.771    1738.271
-----------------------------------------------------------




. svy: total inj_day
(running total on estimation sample)

Survey: Total estimation

Number of strata =        1        Number of obs    =      12
Number of PSUs    =       2        Population size  =      60
                                   Design df        =       1
```

```
-----------------------------------------------------------------
          |              Linearized
          |    Total    Std. Err.       [95% Conf. Interval]
----------+------------------------------------------------------
  inj_day |   1.666667    .745356        -7.80398     11.13731
-----------------------------------------------------------------
```

The estimated total number of visitors per day is 245 and the 95% confidence interval is 0 to 1738. The estimated total number of injuries per day is 1.7 and the 95% confidence interval is 0 to 11.1.

e.   *The number of injuries per visitor.*

Solution:

```
. svy: ratio  injuries visitors
(running ratio on estimation sample)

Survey: Ratio estimation

Number of strata =        1         Number of obs    =      12
Number of PSUs   =        2         Population size  =      60
                                    Design df        =       1

    _ratio_1: injuries/visitors

-----------------------------------------------------------------
          |              Linearized
          |    Ratio    Std. Err.       [95% Conf. Interval]
----------+------------------------------------------------------
 _ratio_1 |   .0068097    .000225        .0039507      .0096687
-----------------------------------------------------------------
```

The estimated number of injuries per visitor is 0.007 and the 95% confidence interval is 0.004 to 0.010.

10.6 *From the population shown in Exercise 10.4, compute the intraclass correlation coefficient for the number of visitors to the park.*

Solution: The intraclass correlation coefficient can be calculated using Equation 10.10.

$$\delta_x = \frac{\frac{1}{\bar{N}}\sigma_{1x}^2 - \sigma_x^2}{(\bar{N}-1)\sigma_x^2}$$

Where σ_{1x}^2 = variance among clusters and σ_{2x}^2 = total variance in x.

These variances can be calculated in STATA. First, the overall variance will be calculated.

```
. sum Visitors

    Variable |      Obs        Mean    Std. Dev.       Min        Max
-------------+-----------------------------------------------------------
    Visitors |       60         208    97.47716         95        495

. display 97.47716^2*59/60
9343.4334
```

Next, the between cluster variance will be calculated. First, the total number of visitors has to be calculated for each cluster. Then, the variance can be calculated.

```
. list Week total

         Week      total
  1.        1        960
  2.        2        680
  3.        3       1153
  4.        4        746
  5.        5        802
  6.        6       1319
  7.        7       2050
  8.        8       2257
  9.        9        906
 10.       10       1607
```

```
. sum total

    Variable |      Obs        Mean    Std. Dev.       Min        Max
-------------+-----------------------------------------------------------
       total |       10        1248    555.5462        680       2257

. display 555.5462^2*9/10
277768.42
```

Finally, calculate the intraclass correlation coefficient.

```
. display ((1/6)*277758.42 - 9343.4334) / (5*9343.4334)
```

10.7   *Using the intraclass correlation coefficient calculated in Exercise 10.6 and assuming* $C_1^* = 2\ _2$, *what would be the optimal number of days to sample in a two-stage cluster sample with weeks as clusters?*

Solution: Equation 10.9 will be used to calculate the optimal number of days to sample in a two-stage cluster sample.

$$\bar{n} = \left[\left(\frac{C_1^*}{C_2^*}\right)\left(\frac{1-\delta_x}{\delta_x}\right)\right]^{\frac{1}{2}} = \left[\left(\frac{100}{40}\right)\left(\frac{1-0.35}{0.35}\right)\right]^{\frac{1}{2}} = 0.727\ or\ 1$$

10.8   *A manufacturer of an orthopedic device would like to initiate a quality control program in which a sample of these devices would be sampled and tested for defects. After the units exit the assembly, they are grouped in batches of 20 boxes, with each box containing 10 units. It is desired to sample each batch and to reject the batch if the estimated proportion of defective units within the batch is above 5%. A pilot study was conducted in which all units within a batch were tested, and the results of this pilot are shown opposite:*

Box	Proportion of Defective Units
1	0.5
2	0.0
3	0.0
4	0.4
5	0.0
6	0.0
7	0.0
8	0.0
9	0.0
10	0.0
11	0.0
12	0.1
13	0.1
14	0.0
15	0.0
16	0.0
17	0.0
18	0.1
19	0.0
20	0.0

Suppose that a two-stage cluster sampling plan were to be used with boxes serving as clusters, and that five units would be selected within each box. Based on the data shown above, how many boxes should be sampled in order that the specifications stated above, be met with 95% confidence.

Solution: To calculate the number of clusters that should be selected, Equation 10.6 will be used.

$$m = \frac{\left(\frac{\sigma_{1x}^2}{\bar{X}^2}\right)*\left(\frac{M}{M-1}\right) + \left(\frac{1}{\bar{n}}\right)*\left(\frac{\sigma_{2x}^2}{\bar{\bar{X}}^2}\right)*\left(\frac{\bar{N}-\bar{n}}{\bar{N}-1}\right)}{\frac{\varepsilon^2}{1.96^2} + \frac{\sigma_{1x}^2}{\bar{X}^2(M-1)}}$$

Let $M = 20, \bar{N} = 10, \bar{n} = 5, \bar{x} = \frac{12}{20} = 0.60, and\ \bar{\bar{x}} = \frac{12}{200} = 0.06.$

$$\hat{\sigma}_{1x}^2 = \frac{\Sigma_{i=1}^m(x_i - \bar{x})^2}{m} = \frac{(5-0.6)^2 + 15(0-0.6)^2 + (4-0.6)^2 + 3(1-0.6)^2}{20}$$
$$= 1.84$$

$$\hat{\sigma}_{2x}^2 = \frac{\Sigma_{i=1}^m \Sigma_{j=1}^{\bar{N}}(x_{ij} - \bar{\bar{x}})^2}{N}$$
$$= \frac{5(0-0.5)^2 + 5(1-0.5)^2 + 15(0-0)^2 + 6(0-0.4)^2 + 4(1-0.4)^2 + 27(0-0.1)^2 + 3(1-0.1)^2}{200}$$
$$= 0.038$$

$$m = \frac{\left(\frac{1.84}{0.60^2}\right)*\left(\frac{20}{19}\right) + \left(\frac{1}{5}\right)*\left(\frac{0.038}{0.06^2}\right)*\left(\frac{10-5}{9}\right)}{\frac{0.05^2}{1.96^2} + \frac{1.84}{0.6^2(19)}} = \frac{5.3801 + 1.173}{0.00065 + 0.2690}$$
$$= 24.31$$

Thus, the specifications cannot be met because over 20 clusters would have to be selected.

10.9   *If in Exercise 10.8, the cost associated with testing the units were 15 times that associated with listing and sampling the boxes, how many units should be sampled within each selected box?*

Solution: To calculate the number of units that should be sampled within each selected box, Equation 10.9 will be used.

$$\bar{n} = \left[\left(\frac{C_1^*}{C_2^*} \right) \left(\frac{1 - \delta_x}{\delta_x} \right) \right]^{1/2}$$

$$\delta_x = \frac{\left(\frac{1}{\bar{N}} \right) \sigma_{1x}^2 - \sigma_x^2}{(\bar{N} - 1)\sigma_x^2} = \frac{\left(\frac{1}{10} \right) 1.84 - \hat{p}(1 - \hat{p})}{(10 - 1)\hat{p}(1 - \hat{p})} = \frac{(0.1)1.84 - 0.6(0.94)}{(9)(0.6)(0.94)}$$
$$= 0.2514$$

$$n = \left[\left(\frac{1}{15} \right) \left(\frac{1 - 0.2514}{0.2514} \right) \right]^{1/2} = 0.4456 \; or \; 1$$

10.10   *Would the data shown in Exercise 10.8 indicate a high or a low intraclass correlation coefficient? State the reason for your answer and verify it by computing the intraclass correlation coefficient.*

Solution: The intraclass correlation coefficient is a measure of how similar the elements within each cluster are. When the elements within each cluster are diverse, the intraclass correlation coefficient will be small because the numerator will be close to zero. The coefficient will be large when the elements within each cluster are homogeneous. I would expect the intraclass correlation coefficient to be larger than zero because the elements within each box tend to be alike: 15 boxes did not contain defective items, 3 contained only one defective item, and the other two had 4 and 5 defective items. Thus, the majority of clusters are very homogeneous.

The intraclass correlation coefficient was calculated in Exercise 10.9 and it is 0.2514. This is larger than zero, as was expected.

10.11 *A study was initiated having as a major objective estimation of the number of patients with severe trauma seen during the calendar year 2004 in hospitals not designated as trauma centers in urban counties in Illinois outside of the Chicago area which have both Trauma Centers (T) and hospitals not designated as Trauma Centers (NT). The following data were available to the investigators:*

County	Hospital	No. of Beds	Type
1	1	310	NT
	2	229	T
	3	367	NT
2	1	134	T
	2	198	NT
3	1	242	T
	2	300	NT
4	1	358	T
	2	410	NT
5	1	32	NT
	2	156	T
6	1	231	NT
	2	209	T
	3	44	NT
7	1	227	NT
	2	178	T
	3	61	NT
	4	59	NT
	5	223	NT
8	1	16	NT
	2	263	T
	3	295	NT
9	1	180	T
	2	152	NT
	3	256	NT
10	1	100	T
	2	65	NT
11	1	595	NT
	2	648	T
12	1	76	NT
	2	133	T
	3	117	NT
	4	117	NT
	5	254	NT
13	1	574	NT
	2	824	T
	3	304	NT
14	1	350	NT
	2	256	T

	3	275	NT
	4	150	NT
15	1	133	NT
	2	314	T
	3	124	T
	4	188	NT
	5	212	NT
	6	143	NT
16	1	60	NT
	2	55	T
17	1	150	T
	2	50	NT
18	1	72	NT
	2	80	T
	3	38	NT
19	1	64	NT
	2	125	T
20	1	367	NT
	2	329	T
	3	312	T
	4	178	NT
	5	281	NT

A two-stage cluster sampling design with counties as primary sampling units and non-trauma center hospitals as listing units was chosen. Six counties were selected at the first stage and one non-trauma center hospital within each sample county was sampled at the second stage. The following data were obtained from this sample survey.

County	Hospital	Cases of Severe Trauma
1	1	14
7	5	10
14	1	6
15	6	0
19	1	1
20	1	24

Use a ratio estimate based on number of beds to estimate from the above sample the total number of cases of severe trauma among hospitals in these 20 counties not designated as trauma centers.

Solution: The equations contained in Box 10.4 in the book will be used for this estimation. Let $N = 39$, $M = 20$, $m = 6$, and $Y = 7844$. We have to weight each sample cluster totals by the number of non-trauma center hospitals in the county.

$$x'_{clu} = \left(\frac{M}{m}\right) * \sum_{i=1}^{m} \left(\frac{N_i}{n_i}\right) \sum_{j=1}^{n_i} x_{ij}$$
$$= \left(\frac{20}{6}\right)[(2*14)+(4*10)+(3*6)+(4*0)+(1*1)+(3*24)] = 530$$

$$y'_{clu} = \left(\frac{M}{m}\right) * \sum_{i=1}^{m} \left(\frac{N_i}{n_i}\right) \sum_{j=1}^{n_i} y_{ij}$$
$$= \left(\frac{20}{6}\right)[(2*310)+(4*223)+(3*350)+(4*143)+(1*64)+(3*367)] = 14,330$$

$$x''_{clu} = \frac{Y}{y'}x' = \frac{7844}{14,330}530 = 290.11 \approx 290$$

10.12 *A sample survey of patient records is being planned in a city that has 25 local mental health centers. The objective of the survey is to estimate the total number of patients who were given diazepam (Valium) as part of their therapeutic regimen. The number of patients treated in each of the mental health centers is listed in the accompanying table. A sample of patients is to be selected by choosing a simple random sample of mental health centers and, within each sample mental health center, choosing a subsample of patients.*

Health Center	No. of Patients	Health Center	No. of Patients
1	491	14	672
2	866	15	475
3	188	16	439
4	994	17	392
5	209	18	584
6	961	19	882
7	834	20	424
8	9,820	21	775
9	348	22	262
10	246	23	968
11	399	24	586
12	175	25	809
13	166		

A survey of 10% of all patients conducted the previous year in health centers 1, 3, 8, 12, and 15 yielded the following data:

Health Center	No. of Patients	No. Given Diazepam
1	46	14
3	13	5
8	94	340
12	15	1
15	42	20

a.   *Based on the data for these five health centers, calculate the intraclass correlation coefficient with respect to the number of patients given diazepam.*

Solution: To calculate the intraclass correlation coefficient from this sample of 5 clusters, Equation 10.20 will be used.

$$\delta_x = \frac{\left[M/(M-1)\right]\sigma_{1x}^2 - \bar{N}\sigma_{2x}^2}{\left[M/(M-1)\right]\sigma_{1x}^2 + \bar{N}(\bar{N}-1)\sigma_{2x}^2}$$

Let $M = 25, m = 5, f_1 = \frac{5}{25},$ and $f_2 =$
   0.10. *We have to estimate* σ_{1x}^2 *and* σ_{2x}^2 *from the sample.*

$$\hat{\sigma}_{1x}^2 = \frac{\sum_{i=1}^m \left(\hat{X}_i - \hat{\bar{X}}\right)^2}{m-1} * \left[\frac{M-1}{M}\right]$$

$$\text{where } \hat{X}_1 = \frac{x_i}{f_2} = 10x_i \text{ and } \hat{\bar{X}} = \frac{\sum_{i=1}^m \hat{X}_i}{m}$$

$$\sigma_{1x}^2 = \frac{(140 - 760)^2 + (50 - 760)^2 + (3400 - 760)^2 + (10 - 760)^2 + (200 - 760)^2}{4}$$

$$* \left[\frac{25-1}{25}\right] = \frac{384,400 + 504,100 + 6,969,600 + 562,500 + 313,600}{4} * \left[\frac{24}{25}\right]$$
$$= 2,096,208$$

$$\sigma_{2x}^2 = \left(\frac{1}{N}\right) \sum_{i=1}^M \left(\frac{N_i}{N_i - 1}\right) \sum_{j=1}^{N_i} (X_{ij} - \bar{X}_i)^2, \text{ where } X_{ij}$$
$$= 1 \text{ if valium is used, } 0 \text{ if not used}$$
$$= \left(\frac{1}{N}\right) \sum_{i=1}^M \left(\frac{N_i}{N_i - 1}\right) N_i (P_i)(1 - P_i)$$

σ_{2x}^2 *can be estimated by* $\sigma_{2x}^2 = \left(\frac{1}{\hat{N}}\right)\left(\frac{M}{m}\right) \sum_{i=1}^M \left(\frac{\hat{N}_i}{\hat{N}_i - 1}\right) \hat{N}_i(\hat{P}_i)(1 - \hat{P}_i)$

$$\text{where } \hat{N} = \frac{\sum_{i=1}^m n_i}{f_2} = 52,900, \bar{N} = \frac{52,900}{25} = 2116, \hat{N}_t = \frac{n_i}{f_2}, \hat{P}_t = \frac{x_i}{n_i} = \frac{\hat{X}_i}{\hat{N}_i}$$

$$\hat{\sigma}_{2x}^2 = \left(\frac{1}{52,900}\right)\left(\frac{25}{5}\right)\left(\frac{460^2}{459} 0.212 + \frac{130^2}{129} 0.237 + \frac{9420^2}{9419} 0.231 + \frac{150^2}{149} 0.063\right.$$
$$\left. + \frac{420^2}{419} 0.249\right)$$
$$= \left(\frac{1}{52,900}\right)\left(\frac{25}{5}\right)(97.73 + 31.05 + 2176.25 + 9.51 + 104.83)$$
$$= \left(\frac{1}{52,900}\right) * 5 * 2419.37 = 0.229$$

$$\delta_x = \frac{\left(\frac{25}{24}\right)(2{,}096{,}208) - (2116)(0.229)}{\left(\frac{25}{24}\right)(2{,}096{,}208) + (2116)(2115)(0.229)} = \frac{2{,}183{,}065.4}{3{,}208{,}402.9}$$

$$= 0.680$$

b.   *Based on the above calculated intraclass correlation coefficient, what would be the optimal average cluster size $\bar{n}$ for the proposed survey of the 25 health centers listed above if the cost component associated with clusters is one thousand times that associated with listing units?*

Solution: Equation 10.22 will be used to calculate the optimal average cluster size.

$$\bar{n} = \left[\left(\frac{C_1}{C_2}\right)\left(\frac{1 - \delta_x}{\delta_x}\right)\right]^{1/2} = \left[\left(\frac{1000}{1}\right)\left(\frac{1 - 0.68}{0.68}\right)\right]^{1/2} = 21.7 \text{ or } 22$$

10.13   *Based on the average cluster size calculated above, how many health centers should be sampled if one wishes to be 95% certain of estimating the number of patients given diazepam to within 10% of the true value?*

Solution: Equation 10.16 will be used to calculate the number of clusters that should be sampled.

$$\text{Let } M = 25, \bar{N} = 2116, \bar{x} = 760, \bar{\bar{x}} = \frac{3800}{10{,}580} = 0.3592, z = 1.96 \text{ and } \varepsilon$$

$$= 0.1.$$

$$m = \frac{\left(\frac{\sigma_{1x}^2}{\bar{X}^2}\right) * \left(\frac{M}{M-1}\right) + \left(\frac{M}{N^2\bar{\bar{X}}^2}\right) * \left[\sum_{i=1}^{m}\left(\frac{N_i}{n_i}\right)\left(\frac{N_i - n_i}{N_i - 1}\right)\left(\sum_{j-1}^{N_i}(X_{ij} - \bar{X}_i)^2\right)\right]}{\frac{\varepsilon^2}{1.96^2} + \frac{\sigma_{1x}^2}{\bar{X}^2(M-1)}}$$

$$\text{where } \sum_{j-1}^{N_i}(X_{ij} - \bar{X}_i)^2 = \sum_{i=1}^{m} N_i P_i(1 - P_i)$$

$$\text{Let } A = \left(\frac{M}{N^2\bar{\bar{X}}^2}\right) * \left[\sum_{i=1}^{m}\left(\frac{N_i}{n_i}\right)\left(\frac{N_i - n_i}{N_i - 1}\right)\sum_{i=1}^{m} N_i P_i(1 - P_i)\right]$$

We can estimate A using Â

$$\hat{A} = \left(\frac{M}{\widehat{N}^2\hat{\bar{X}}^2}\right) * \left[\frac{M}{m}\sum_{i=1}^{m}\left(\frac{\widehat{N}_i}{n_i}\right)\left(\frac{\widehat{N}_i - n_i}{N_i - 1}\right)\sum_{i=1}^{m}\widehat{N}_i\widehat{P}_i(1 - \widehat{P}_i)\right]$$

$$\widehat{N} = \frac{M}{m}\sum_{i=1}^{m}\widehat{N}_i \ and \ \widehat{N}_i = \frac{n_i}{f_2},$$

$$\widehat{X} = \frac{M}{m}\sum_{i=1}^{m}\widehat{X}_i \ and \ \widehat{X}_i = \frac{x_i}{f_2},$$

$$\hat{\bar{X}} = \frac{\widehat{X}}{N} = \frac{19,000}{52,900} = 0.359$$

$$\widehat{P}_i = \frac{x_i}{m_i}$$

$$\hat{A} = \frac{25}{52,900^2 * 0.359^2}\left[\frac{25}{5}(877.866 + 279.174 + 19,559.042 + 84.956 \right.$$
$$\left. + 945.073)\right] = 0.00754$$

$$m = \frac{\left(\frac{2,096,208}{760^2}\right) * \left(\frac{25}{24}\right) + 0.00754}{\frac{0.1^2}{1.96^2} + \frac{2,096,208}{760^2 * 24}} = \frac{3.780 + 0.00754}{0.0026 + 0.1512} = \frac{3.78754}{0.1538}$$
$$= 24.62 \ or \ 25$$

10.14   *What would be the standard error of the estimated total number of patients given diazepam based on the cluster size n and number m of sample clusters determined in Exercises 10.12 and 10.13?*

Solution: For this problem, we will assume the sample data were obtained using simple random sampling in order to calculate σ_x.

$$\sigma_x = \sqrt{pq}$$

$$where\ p = \frac{380}{1058} = 0.359$$

$$\sigma_x = \sqrt{0.359(1 - 0.359)} = 0.4798$$

$$SE(x'_{clu}) = \frac{\hat{N}\sigma_x}{\sqrt{n}}\sqrt{1 + \delta_x(\bar{n} - 1)} = \frac{52{,}900 * 0.4798}{\sqrt{22 * 25}}\sqrt{1 + 0.680(22 - 1)}$$
$$= 1082.267 * 3.909 = 4230.58$$

10.15   *A household survey is to be conducted for purposes of estimating certain health status and health utilization variables. The survey research laboratory contracted to perform the study has access to U.S. Census Bureau lists of households and can define clusters of 18 households from which a sample of households can be taken. From a study conducted on similar lists the intraclass correlation coefficients were estimate (see the accompanying table). It estimated that the cost component associated with clusters is about one-fourth of that associated with listing units. On the basis of this information, choose between the three different types of clusters and determine the appropriate sample cluster size.*

	Intraclass Correlation for Various Cluster Sizes		
Variable	*$N_i = 6$*	*$N_i = 9$*	*$N_i = 18$*
Number of bed-days in last 2 weeks	*0.022*	*0.038*	*0.011*
Number of hospital discharges in past 12 months	*0.057*	*0.069*	*0.077*

Solution: For each cluster size, the sample cluster size will be estimated for both the number of bed-days and number of discharges. The average of the two will then be calculated. The cluster size that minimizes the sample size will be chosen because the greatest cost is associated with the listing units. Thus, the goal is to minimize the number of listing units sampled in each cluster.

	Optimal Sample Size for each Cluster Size		
Variable	$N_i = 6$	$N_i = 9$	$N_i = 18$
Number of bed-days in last 2 weeks	3.33	2.52	4.74
Number of hospital discharges in past 12 months	2.03	1.84	1.73
Average of two	2.68	2.18	3.24

On the basis of the above results, the cluster size $N_i = 9$ should be chosen because it minimizes, for a given total sample size, the number of listing units that have to be sampled.

10.16 *A list of hospitals in a rural geographic area is shown in the accompanying table, by county. A sample survey is planned using a sample design in which counties are clusters, hospitals are listing units, and one hospital is to be selected from each county. If it is assumed that the total expenses for a hospital are proportional to the number of admissions, how many counties should be selected in order to b e 95% confident of estimating the total expenses per day among hospitals in that region to within 20% of the true value?*

County	Hospital	No. of Beds	Average No. of Admissions per Day in 1989
1	1	72	4.8
2	1	87	8.4
	2	104	9.4
	3	34	2.0
3	1	99	5.1
4	1	48	4.4
5	1	99	6.2
6	1	131	9.1
	2	182	15.9
7	1	42	2.4
8	1	38	2.8
9	1	34	2.3
10	1	42	4.9
11	1	39	4.0
	2	59	4.1
12	1	76	5.2
13	1	25	3.1
	2	80	5.3
14	1	50	4.9
15	1	88	7.1
16	1	50	4.4
17	1	63	5.1
18	1	45	3.9
19	1	75	8.5
20	1	17	3.8
	2	140	11.9
21	1	44	4.9
22	1	171	12.0
	2	85	4.6
23	1	48	3.8
	2	18	2.9
24	1	54	4.9
25	1	68	3.8
	2	68	5.5
26	1	44	3.5
27	1	32	1.0
	2	90	6.1
28	1	35	2.9
29	1	72	5.2
30	1	104	6.6
31	1	86	6.4
	2	91	6.4
	3	53	4.5
32	1	108	6.4
33	1	50	4.9
34	1	45	3.8
35	1	65	4.3
36	1	48	4.9
37	1	61	5.7

Solution: Equation 10.16 will be used to estimate the sample size.

Let $M = 37, \bar{n} = 1, z = 1.96, and\ \varepsilon = 0.20$

$$m = \frac{\left(\frac{\sigma_{1x}^2}{\bar{X}^2}\right)*\left(\frac{M}{M-1}\right)+\left(\frac{M}{N^2\bar{\bar{X}}^2}\right)*\left[\sum_{i=1}^{m}\left(\frac{N_i}{n_i}\right)\left(\frac{N_i-n_i}{N_i-1}\right)\left(\sum_{j-1}^{N_i}(X_{ij}-\bar{\bar{X}}_i)^2\right)\right]}{\frac{\varepsilon^2}{1.96^2}+\frac{\sigma_{1x}^2}{\bar{X}^2(M-1)}}$$

In STATA we can estimate the variance among the clusters. First, create a file that contains the county number and the average number of admissions within each cluster.

```
. list

      county   admissns
 1.      1       4.8
 2.      2       6.6
 3.      3       5.1
 4.      4       4.4
 5.      5       6.2
 6.      6      12.5
 7.      7       2.4
 8.      8       2.8
 9.      9       2.3
10.     10       4.9
11.     11       4.1
12.     12       5.2
13.     13       4.2
14.     14       4.9
15.     15       7.1
16.     16       4.4
17.     17       5.1
18.     18       3.9
19.     19       8.5
20.     20       7.9
21.     21       4.9
22.     22       8.3
23.     23       3.4
24.     24       4.9
25.     25       4.7
26.     26       3.5
27.     27       3.6
28.     28       2.9
29.     29       5.2
30.     30       6.6
31.     31       5.8
32.     32       6.4
33.     33       4.9
34.     34       3.8
35.     35       4.3
36.     36       4.9
37.     37       5.7
```

Next, calculate the variance among clusters.

```
. sum admissns, detail

                            Admissns
-------------------------------------------------------------
          Percentiles     Smallest
    1%        2.3            2.3
    5%        2.4            2.4
   10%        2.9            2.8        Obs                  37
   25%        4.1            2.9        Sum of Wgt.          37

   50%        4.9                       Mean           5.164865
                            Largest     Std. Dev.      1.947394
   75%        5.8            7.9
   90%        7.9            8.3        Variance       3.792342
   95%        8.5            8.5        Skewness       1.554571
   99%       12.5           12.5        Kurtosis       6.776546

. display 3.792342 * (4/5)
3.0338736
```

The within cluster variance is calculated next. Only counties with more than one hospital contribute to the variance (counties 2, 6, 11, 13, 20, 22, 23, 25, 27, and 31).

$$\sum_{i=1}^{m} \left(\frac{N_i}{n_i}\right)\left(\frac{N_i - n_i}{N_i - 1}\right)\left(\sum_{j-1}^{N_i}(X_{ij} - \bar{\bar{X}}_i)^2\right)$$

$$= \left(\frac{3}{1} * \frac{3-1}{3-1} * (3.24 + 7.84 + 32.24)\right) + \left(\frac{2}{1} * \frac{2-1}{2-1} * 2(11.56)\right)$$

$$+ \left(\frac{2}{1} * \frac{2-1}{2-1} * 2(0.0025)\right) + \left(\frac{2}{1} * \frac{2-1}{2-1} * 2(1.21)\right)$$

$$+ \left(\frac{2}{1} * \frac{2-1}{2-1} * 2(16.403)\right) + \left(\frac{2}{1} * \frac{2-1}{2-1} * 2(13.69)\right)$$

$$+ \left(\frac{2}{1} * \frac{2-1}{2-1} * 2(0.23)\right) + \left(\frac{2}{1} * \frac{2-1}{2-1} * 2(0.723)\right)$$

$$+ \left(\frac{2}{1} * \frac{2-1}{2-1} * 2(6.503)\right) + \left(\frac{3}{1} * \frac{3-1}{3-1} * (0.397 + 0.397 + 1.61)\right)$$

$$= 129.96 + 46.24 + 0.01 + 4.84 + 65.612 + 54.76 + 0.92 + 2.892$$

$$+ 26.012 + 7.221 = 338.467$$

$$m = \frac{\left(\frac{\sigma_{1x}^2}{\bar{X}^2}\right)*\left(\frac{M}{M-1}\right)+\left(\frac{M}{N^2\bar{\bar{X}}^2}\right)*\left[\sum_{i=1}^{m}\left(\frac{N_i}{n_i}\right)\left(\frac{N_i-n_i}{N_i-1}\right)\left(\sum_{j-1}^{N_i}(X_{ij}-\bar{\bar{X}}_i)^2\right)\right]}{\frac{\varepsilon^2}{1.96^2}+\frac{\sigma_{1x}^2}{\bar{X}^2(M-1)}}$$

$$=\frac{\left(\frac{3.034}{5.165^2}\right)*\left(\frac{37}{36}\right)+\left(\frac{37}{49^2*5.388^2}\right)338.467}{\frac{0.2^2}{1.96^2}+\frac{3.034}{5.165^2(36)}}=\frac{0.117+0.180}{0.010+0.003}=\frac{0.297}{0.013}$$

$$= 22.8 \text{ or } 23$$

10.17 Suppose that a simple random sample of five clusters is selected from the population shown in Exercise 10.16 and that the clusters selected are 5, 8, 23, 30, and 36. Take a second-stage sample of 1 listing unit from each sample cluster and estimate from this sample the mean number of admissions per hospital bed. (Use statistical software if available.)

Solution: STATA will be used to estimate the mean number of admissions per hospital bed. Hospital 2 in cluster 23 was selected for this sample.

```
. gen M = 37

. gen wt = M / 5

. replace wt = (M / 5) * (2 / 1) if county == 23
(1 real change made)

. svyset county [pweight=wt]
      pweight: wt
          VCE: linearized
  Single unit: missing
     Strata 1: <one>
        SU 1: county
       FPC 1: <zero>

. svy: ratio admissns beds
(running ratio on estimation sample)

Survey: Ratio estimation

Number of strata =        1      Number of obs    =        5
Number of PSUs   =        5      Population size  =     44.4
                                 Design df        =        4

    _ratio_1: admissns/beds

------------------------------------------------------------
             |             Linearized
             |     Ratio   Std. Err.   [95% Conf. Interval]
-------------+----------------------------------------------
   _ratio_1 |  .0809231   .0137689     .0426945    .1191516
------------------------------------------------------------
```

The sample mean number of admissions per hospital bed is 0.01. A 95% confidence interval for this estimate is 0.04 to 0.12.

10.18   From the sample taken in Exercise 10.17 estimate the total number of admissions for 2008 among the 37 counties in this region. What is the estimated standard error of this estimate? (Use appropriate statistical software if available.)

Solution: STATA will be used to obtain the estimated total number of admissions for 1989, and the standard error of this estimate.

```
. gen adm_yr = admissns * 365

. svy: total adm_yr
(running total on estimation sample)

Survey: Total estimation

Number of strata =        1        Number of obs   =       5
Number of PSUs   =        5        Population size  =    44.4
                                   Design df        =       4

------------------------------------------------------------
            |                 Linearized
            |     Total    Std. Err.     [95% Conf. Interval]
------------+-----------------------------------------------
     adm_yr |   71036.3   9135.611      45671.78   96400.82
------------------------------------------------------------
```

The estimated total number of admissions in 1989 for these 37 counties is 71,036 and the standard error of this estimate is 9135.6. A 95% confidence interval is 45,572 to 96,400. From the population data, the total number of admissions is 96,360. Thus, the 95% confidence just covers the true population value.

10.19 *A simple random sample of five gasoline stations was taken in a medium-size city containing 30 such stations. Within each of these five sample stations, a mobile unit with equipment to collect urine and saliva specimens was set up, and a sample of 1 in 10 automobiles entering the station was taken. The driver of each sampled automobile was requested to participate in the survey which consisted of a short interview and submission of a urine and saliva specimen. Each participant was given a free tank of gasoline as an incentive and assured that the information obtained was strictly confidential. The major objective of the survey was to obtain estimates of the number of drivers who show evidence of substance abuse while driving. The following data were obtained:*

Station	Number of Persons Tested	Number of Persons Showing Evidence of Substance Abuse
1	15	3
2	6	1
3	11	1
4	6	3
5	8	1

a. *Based on these data, estimate the number of drivers in the city who show evidence of substance abuse.*

Solution: First, create a file in STATA that contains the station number and the results from each person's test.

```
. list

       station    abuse     wt
 1.       1         1        60
 2.       1         1        60
 3.       1         1        60
 4.       1         0        60
 5.       1         0        60
 6.       1         0        60
 7.       1         0        60
 8.       1         0        60
 9.       1         0        60
10.       1         0        60
11.       1         0        60
12.       1         0        60
13.       1         0        60
14.       1         0        60
15.       1         0        60
16.       2         1        60
17.       2         0        60
18.       2         0        60
19.       2         0        60
20.       2         0        60
21.       2         0        60
22.       3         1        60
23.       3         0        60
24.       3         0        60
25.       3         0        60
26.       3         0        60
27.       3         0        60
28.       3         0        60
29.       3         0        60
30.       3         0        60
31.       3         0        60
32.       3         0        60
33.       4         1        60
34.       4         1        60
35.       4         1        60
36.       4         0        60
37.       4         0        60
38.       4         0        60
39.       5         1        60
40.       5         0        60
41.       5         0        60
42.       5         0        60
43.       5         0        60
44.       5         0        60
45.       5         0        60
46.       5         0        60
```

Next, use the svy: total procedure in STATA to obtain the estimated total number of drivers in the city who show evidence of substance abuse.

```
. gen wt = (30 / 5) * (10 / 1)

. svyset station [pweight=wt]

      pweight: wt
          VCE: linearized
  Single unit: missing
     Strata 1: <one>
         SU 1: station
        FPC 1: <zero>

. svy: total  abuse
(running total on estimation sample)

Survey: Total estimation

Number of strata =         1      Number of obs   =       46
Number of PSUs   =         5      Population size =     2760
                                  Design df       =        4


----------------------------------------------------------------
               |              Linearized
               |     Total    Std. Err.     [95% Conf. Interval]
---------------+------------------------------------------------
         abuse |       540    146.9694       131.9476    948.0524
----------------------------------------------------------------
```

The estimated total is 540 and the 95% confidence interval is 132 to 948.

b.   *Is the estimate used above unbiased? Show that it is/is not.*

Solution: In the second stage, a systematic sample was taken. We do not know the number of drivers that actually were counted at each station, that is, the N_i. If $N_i/10$ is not an integer, then the estimate is biased. The refusal rate should also be considered, and this was not mentioned in the problem. People who refuse to participate may be more or less likely to be substance abusers than those who agreed to participate. We should also consider the driver's total time on the road and the gas mileage of his/her vehicle. This could impact on the likelihood of the driver appearing at the gas station.

c.   *If it is not unbiased, what further information would be needed to construct an unbiased estimate?*

Solution: We need the N_i, or total number of drivers counted at each station.

Chapter Eleven – Solutions

11.1 Let us consider again the population of 25 local mental health centers of Exercises 10.12-10.15 (table reproduced here):

Health Center	No. of Patients	Health Center	No. of Patients
1	491	14	672
2	866	15	475
3	188	16	439
4	994	17	392
5	209	18	584
6	961	19	882
7	834	20	424
8	9,820	21	775
9	348	22	262
10	246	23	968
11	399	24	586
12	175	25	809
13	166		

Suppose that you wish to take a two-stage PPS sample with replacement of health centers for purposes of estimating the total number of patients currently taking Prozac. Suppose further that the measure of size variable for the PPS sampling is the number of patients, and that the random numbers chosen are 11,052 and 12,614.

a.   *Which two health centers are sampled?*

Solution: Health center 8 is sampled twice.

b.   *Suppose that a simple random sample of 20 patients is taken at each drawing from the health center selected at that drawing. Suppose further that the sample corresponding to the random number, 11,052, contains 12 patients on Prozac, and that the sample corresponding to the random number, 12,614, contains 6 persons on Prozac. Use the Hansen-Hurwitz estimator to estimate the total number of persons on Prozac. What is the estimated standard error of that estimate?*

Solution: Equation 10.9 in the text will be used to estimate the total number of persons on Prozac and Equation 11.10 will be used to estimate the standard error. Let $m = 2$, $N_1 = N_2 = 9820$, $N = 22,965$, and $n = 40$.

$$y'_{ppswr} = \frac{N}{n}\sum_{i=1}^{m} y_i = \frac{22,965}{40}(12+6) = 10,334.25$$

$$\widehat{SE}(y'_{ppswr}) = \sqrt{\frac{\sum_{i=1}^{m}\left(\frac{N_i X y_i}{\bar{n} X_i} - y'_{ppswr}\right)^2}{m(m-1)}}$$

$$= \sqrt{\frac{(13,779 - 10,335.25)^2 + (6889.5 - 10,334.25)^2}{2}} = 3444.75$$

11.2 It is desired to estimate the number of Koreans living in a particular city. The city encompasses six telephone exchanges, and examination of the latest telephone directory showed the following frequencies of the two most common Korean surnames—Kim and Park.

Exchange	Population of Geographic Area Corresponding to Exchange	No. of Kims and Parks in Directory
832	5231	21
856	3012	8
935	2123	7
936	1256	35
937	2569	17
983	8321	10

It is thought that approximately 60% of all Koreans in that area have either "Kim" or "Park" as surnames, and that the average Korean household comprises four persons.

a. If you were to use exchanges as clusters, what method of sampling the clusters should be used?

Solution: The sampling method that should be used is probably proportional to size sampling, applying more weight to the areas that have a greater proportion of Korean surnames.

b. Use this method to take a sample of three exchanges. Show in detail how the sample was selected.

Solution: The methods outlined in Section 11.3.3 in the text will be used to select this sample. First, the number of Kims and Parks will be cumulated and associated with random numbers within each cluster.

Exchange	Population of Geographic Area Corresponding to Exchange	No. of Kims and Parks in Directory	Cumulative number of Parks and Kims	Random Numbers
832	5231	21	21	01-21
856	3012	8	29	22-29
935	2123	7	36	30-36
936	1256	35	71	37-71
937	2569	17	88	72-88
983	8321	10	98	89-98

Next, select three random numbers between 1 and 98 from Table A.1. Suppose we start with column 3, line 21 and then work down the column. Taking the last two digits of each random number, we would select numbers 28, 21 and 97. These numbers correspond to exchanges 856, 832, and 983.

11.3   *From the population of counties shown in Exercise 10.16, a PPS sample with replacement of 5 counties is taken, and for every selection of a county at the first stage, a sample of 1 hospital is taken at the second stage. The sampling is performed as follows:*

a. The procedure for taking a PPS sample of counties is that described in Section 11.3.3.
b. The measure of size variable for sampling a county is the total number of hospitals within the county.
c. The random numbers chosen for selection of the sample are as follows:

Selection Sequence	Random Number for Selection of Counties at First Stage	Random Number for Selection of Counties at Second Stage
1	38	1
2	24	1
3	24	1
4	42	3
5	08	1

From the above information, determine the sample counties and hospitals.

Solution: Using these procedures, we can complete the table below.

Selection Sequence	Random Number for Selection of Counties at First Stage	Random Number for Selection of Counties at Second Stage	County	Hospital
1	38	1	28	1
2	24	1	19	1
3	24	1	19	1
4	42	3	31	3
5	08	1	6	1

11.4 *From the sample selected in the previous exercise, determine the total number of hospital admissions during 1989 in the 37 county region. Also, determine the standard error of this estimated total.*

Solution: We will use STATA to obtain this estimate and the standard error of the estimate. First, the data will be entered in to the data editor.

```
. list  Selectn County Hospital Adm_day Beds

       Selectn    County  Hospital   Adm_day       Beds
  1.         1        28         1       2.9         35
  2.         2        19         1       8.5         75
  3.         3        19         1       8.5         75
  4.         4        31         3       4.5         53
  5.         5         6         1       9.1        131
```

Next, use the survey procedures in STATA to obtain the desired estimates.

```
. gen wt=49/5

. gen adm=adm_day*365

. svyset  selectn [pweight=wt]

      pweight: wt
          VCE: linearized
 Single unit: missing
    Strata 1: <one>
        SU 1: selectn
       FPC 1: <zero>
```

```
. svy: total adm
(running total on estimation sample)

Survey: Total estimation

Number of strata =        1        Number of obs      =        5
Number of PSUs    =        5        Population size    =       49
                                    Design df          =        4


-----------------------------------------------------------------
                 |                Linearized
                 |     Total      Std. Err.      [95% Conf. Interval]
-----------------+-----------------------------------------------
             adm |    119829.5     22452.62       57491.03      182168
-----------------------------------------------------------------
```

The estimated total number of hospital admissions in the 37 counties is 119,830 and the standard error of this estimate is 22,453. The 95% confidence interval is 57,491 to 182,168.

11.5   *(For those having access to software such as STATA or SUDAAN.) Estimate the total number of admissions per bed from the sample selected in Exercise 11.3. Also, determine the standard error of this estimate.*

Solution: We will use the svy: ratio procedure in STATA to obtain this estimate and the standard error of the estimate.

```
. svy: ratio adm beds
(running ratio on estimation sample)

Survey: Ratio estimation

Number of strata =        1        Number of obs      =        5
Number of PSUs    =        5        Population size    =       49
                                    Design df          =        4

    _ratio_1: adm/beds


-----------------------------------------------------------------
                 |                Linearized
                 |     Ratio      Std. Err.      [95% Conf. Interval]
-----------------+-----------------------------------------------
        _ratio_1 |    33.13686    4.092492       21.77428      44.49944
-----------------------------------------------------------------
```

The estimated total number of admissions per bed is 33.1 and the standard error of this estimate is 4.1. The 95% confidence interval is 21.8 to 44.5.

11.6 *(For those having access to SAS): Download the SAS data file court1.sasbdat from the Wiley FTP. This file contains the data for the 26 district courts discussed in Section 11.3.4. From this file, using PROC SURVEYSELECT in SAS, and using the seed 61420009, take a PMR sample of 12 PSUs. Using the same seed, take a PPS sample with replacement of 12 PSUs. Compare the two samples.*

```
proc surveyselect data=court
      method=pps_seq samplesize=12
      seed=61420009 out=pmr_sample;
      size num_eligible;
      run;

proc surveyselect data=court
      method=pps_seq samplesize=12
      seed=61420009 out=pmr_sample;
      size num_eligible;
      run;
```

Solution: By PMR sampling the following courts were selected:

District Court	Number of Eligible Persons	Number of Hits	Expected Number of Hits	Sampling Weight
24	1398	1	1.0919	0.91583
25	1755	1	1.37074	0.72953
26	1513	2	1.18172	0.84622
4	508	1	0.39677	2.52034
6	486	1	0.37959	2.63443
11	305	1	0.23822	4.19781
17	1130	1	0.88258	1.13304
19	983	1	0.76777	1.30248
22	1506	2	1.17626	0.85015
23	1181	1	0.92242	1.08411

By PPS with Replacement the following courts were selected:

District Court	Number of Eligible Persons	Number of Hits	Expected Number of Hits	Sampling Weight
6	486	2	0.37959	2.63443
10	240	1	0.18745	5.33472
18	1000	1	0.78105	1.28033
19	983	1	0.76777	1.30248
22	1506	2	1.17626	0.85015
23	1181	2	0.92242	1.08411
24	1398	2	1.0919	0.91583
26	1513	1	1.18172	0.84622

Chapter Twelve – Solutions

12.1   *Let $\bar{x}$ be an estimate of the mean level of a variable X, and $\bar{y}$ be an estimate of the mean level of a variable Y, where both are obtained from simple random sampling. Let $\bar{z} = \overline{xy}$. Use linearization to find an expression for the estimated variance of the distribution of $\bar{z}$.*

Solution: Using the procedures outlined in Section 12.1, for subject i, the linearized value is:

$$z_i = (\partial f_{\bar{x}})x_i + (\partial f_{\bar{y}})y_i$$

$$\partial f_{\bar{x}} = \frac{\partial f(\bar{x},\bar{y})}{\partial \bar{x}} \text{ evaluated at point } (\bar{X},\bar{Y})$$

$$\partial f_{\bar{y}} = \frac{\partial f(\bar{x},\bar{y})}{\partial \bar{y}} \text{ evaluated at point } (\bar{X},\bar{Y})$$

In this example,

$$\partial f_{\bar{x}} = \bar{y}$$

$$\partial f_{\bar{y}} = \bar{x}$$

$$z_i = \bar{y}x + \bar{x}y$$

$$\bar{z} = \frac{1}{n}\sum_{i=1}^{n} z_i = \frac{1}{n}\sum_{i=1}^{n}(\bar{y}x_i + \bar{x}y_i)$$

$$Var(\bar{z}) = Var\left(\frac{1}{n}\sum_{i=1}^{n} z_i\right)\left(\frac{N-n}{N-1}\right) = \frac{1}{n^2}Var\left(\sum_{i=1}^{n} z_i\right)\left(\frac{N-n}{N-1}\right)$$

$$= \frac{1}{n^2}\sum_{i-1}^{n} Var(z_i)\left(\frac{N-n}{N-1}\right) = \frac{1}{n^2}*n*Var(z_i)\left(\frac{N-n}{N-1}\right)$$

$$= \frac{1}{n}Var(z_i)\left(\frac{N-n}{N-1}\right) = \frac{1}{n}Var(\bar{y}x_i + \bar{x}y_i)\left(\frac{N-n}{N-1}\right)$$

$$= \frac{1}{n}\{Var(\bar{y}x_i) + Var(\bar{x}y_i) + 2Cov(\bar{y}x_i, \bar{x}y_i)\}\left(\frac{N-n}{N-1}\right)$$

$$= \frac{1}{n}\{\bar{y}^2 Var(x_i) + \bar{x}^2 Var(y_i) + 2\overline{xy}\rho_{xy}\sigma_x\sigma_y\}\left(\frac{N-n}{N-1}\right)$$

$$= \frac{1}{n}\{\bar{y}^2\sigma_x^2 + \bar{x}^2\sigma_y^2 + 2\overline{xy}\rho_{xy}\sigma_x\sigma_y\}\left(\frac{N-n}{N-1}\right)$$

$$= \frac{1}{n}\{\bar{y}^2 V_x^2 \bar{x}^2 + \bar{x}^2 V_y^2 \bar{y}^2 + 2\overline{xy}\rho_{xy}(V_x\bar{x})(V_y\bar{y})\}\left(\frac{N-n}{N-1}\right)$$

$$= \frac{\bar{x}^2\bar{y}^2}{n}\{V_x^2 + V_y^2 + 2\rho V_x V_y\}\left(\frac{N-n}{N-1}\right)$$

12.2   *In a large state there are 34 counties that are not in metropolitan areas. For purposes of estimating the total number of admissions during the calendar year 2000 to hospitals in this 34-county area with acquired immune deficiency syndrome (AIDS), these counties are grouped into six strata, and a simple random sample of two counties is selected within each stratum. Within each of the sample counties, a simple random sample of one hospital is taken, and within each sample hospital, all hospital medical records of patients having a discharge diagnosis of AIDS are reviewed, abstracted, and enumerated. The following table lists the hospitals by stratum, county, and number of beds.*

Stratification for AIDS Admission Survey

Stratum	County	Hospital	Beds
1	1	1	72
1	2	1	87
1	2	2	104
1	2	3	34
1	3	1	17
1	3	2	140
1	4	1	104
2	1	1	44
2	2	1	99
2	3	1	86
2	3	2	91
2	3	3	53
2	4	1	48
3	1	1	171
3	1	2	85
3	2	1	108
3	3	1	99
3	4	1	131
3	4	2	182
4	1	1	48
4	1	2	18
4	2	1	50
4	3	1	42
4	4	1	38
5	1	1	42
5	2	1	54
5	3	1	45
5	4	1	34
6	1	1	39
6	1	2	59
6	2	1	76
6	3	1	68
6	3	2	68
6	4	1	65

a.   *Show how you would estimate the number of AIDS admissions for the 34-county area, taking into consideration number of beds.*

   Solution: We should use a ratio estimate of the total. Using Equation 7.4,

$$x'' = \left(\frac{x'}{y'}\right) * Y$$

b.   *The hospitals actually sampled are shown in the accompanying table along with the number of AIDS admissions enumerated at each sample hospital. From these data, estimate the total number of AIDS admissions for the 34-county areas.*

Hospitals in Sample

Stratum	County	Hospital	Beds	Total AIDS
1	1	1	72	20
1	2	1	87	49
2	2	1	99	38
2	4	1	48	23
3	3	1	99	38
3	4	1	131	78
4	3	1	42	7
4	4	1	38	28
5	1	1	42	26
5	4	1	34	9
6	1	1	39	18
6	2	1	76	20

   Solution: Applying Equation 7.4 to these data, we obtain

$$x'' = \left(\frac{x'}{y'}\right) * Y = \left(\frac{354}{807}\right) * 2501 = 1097.1$$

c.   Use a set of balanced half samples to estimate the standard error of the estimated total number of AIDS admissions for the 34-county area. The following Plackett-Burman matrix can be used to construct the half sample estimates (McCarthy [6, p.17]):

			Stratum			
Rep.	1	2	3	4	5	6
1	+	−	−	+	−	+
2	+	+	−	−	+	−
3	+	+	+	−	−	+
4	+	+	+	+	−	−
5	−	−	+	+	+	−
6	−	+	-	+	+	+
7	−	−	+	−	+	+
8	−	−	−	−	−	−

Solution: The problem will be solved using SUDAAN. The output is shown below. Each of the numbered commands shown below were written into a file and executed.

```
1    PROC RATIO DATA = NEWEX12 FILETYPE=SAS DESIGN=BRR;
2    WEIGHT WT;
3    REPWGT REP1 REP2 REP3 REP4 REP5 REP6 REP7 REP8;
4    NUMER AIDSBEDS;
5    DENOM BEDS;

Opened SAS data file C:\PROGRAM
FILES\SUDAAN\RELEASE801\EXAMPLES\STANDALONE\NEWEX12.SSD for reading.

Number of observations read   :    12    Weighted count :       32
Denominator degrees of freedom :     8


Variance Estimation Method: BRR
by: Variable, One.

---------------------------------------------------
|             |               |               |
| Variable    |               | One           |
|             |               | 1             |
---------------------------------------------------
|             |               |               |
| AIDSBEDS/BEDS | Sample Size  |          12 |
|             | Weighted Size  |       32.00 |
|             | Weighted X-Sum |     2302.00 |
|             | Weighted Y-Sum | 2741096.00 |
|             | Ratio Est.     |     1190.75 |
|             | SE Ratio       |      156.54 |
---------------------------------------------------
```

The estimated total number of AIDS admissions is 1190.75, or 1191. The standard error, estimated using the BRR method, is 156.54.

d.   *Use the jackknife method to obtain the standard error of the estimated total number of AIDS admissions for the 34-county area. Compare this to the BRR estimate obtained in part (c).*

Solution: Again, we will use SUDAAN to solve this problem.

```
6    PROC RATIO DATA = NEWEX12 FILETYPE=SAS DESIGN=JACKKNIFE;
7    NEST STRATUM COUNTY;
8    WEIGHT WT;
9    NUMER AIDSBEDS;

Opened SAS data file C:\PROGRAM
FILES\SUDAAN\RELEASE801\EXAMPLES\STANDALONE\NEWEX12.SSD for reading.
10   DENOM BEDS;

Number of observations read    :    12    Weighted count :        32
Denominator degrees of freedom :     6




Variance Estimation Method: Delete-1 Jackknife
by: Variable, One.


--------------------------------------------------------
|                    |                |                 |
| Variable           |                | One             |
|                    |                | 1               |
--------------------------------------------------------
|                    |                |                 |
| AIDSBEDS/BEDS      | Sample Size    |          12 |
|                    | Weighted Size  |       32.00 |
|                    | Weighted X-Sum |     2302.00 |
|                    | Weighted Y-Sum |  2741096.00 |
|                    | Ratio Est.     |     1190.75 |
|                    | SE Ratio       |      141.34 |
--------------------------------------------------------
```

The estimated total number of AIDS admissions is 1190.75, or 1191. The standard error, estimated using the jackknife method, is 141.34.

Both the BRR and the jackknife methods result in similar estimated totals. The standard error computed using the jackknife method is smaller than the one computed using the BRR method.

Note: There are 24 counties and 34 hospitals in the target population, not 34 counties as stated in several places in the exercise.

12.3 *A sample survey of video stores was taken for purposes of estimating the proportion of these stores that offer incentives to customers based on prepaid membership plans. A simple random sample of 48 such establishments was taken and each of 6 interviewers was randomly allocated 8 such stores for a telephone interview. The following data were obtained:*

Interviewer	Number Having Prepaid Membership Plans
1	7
2	1
3	0
4	8
5	7
6	0

Is there evidence of an interviewer effect? If "yes," how great is this effect?

Solution: The procedures outlined in Section 12.2.3 will be used to estimate the interviewer effect.

Let $M = 48, m = 6,$ and $\bar{n} = 8$.

Interviewer	p_i
1	0.875
2	0.125
3	0
4	1.0
5	0.875
6	0

$$s_{bx}^2 = \frac{\bar{n}\sum_{i=1}^{m}(x_i - \bar{x})^2}{m - 1} = \frac{8}{5}(0.3133 + 0.1255 + 0.4593 + 0.2172) = 1.868$$

$$s_{wx}^2 = \sum_{i=1}^{m}\frac{\bar{n}*p_i(1 - p_i)}{m(\bar{n} - 1)} = 0.0625$$

$$\frac{s_{bx}^2}{s_{wx}^2} = 29.88 > F_{5,42}$$

Because the F value is much larger than the critical value, we conclude that there is an interviewer effect. From the calculation below, 78.3 percent of the total variance is explained by the interviewer effect.

$$\delta_x = \frac{\left(\frac{s_{bx}^2}{s_{wx}^2} - 1\right)}{\left(\frac{s_{bx}^2}{s_{wx}^2} - 1 + \bar{n}\right)} = 0.783$$

12.4   Use the jackknife method to estimate the standard error of the overpayment proportion for the data in Table 12.1. How does this compare with that obtained by the linearization method?

Solution: In this problem, SUDAAN will be used to estimate the standard error using the jackknife method. Using the jackknife method, the standard error is estimated to be 0.132. This is larger than the standard error estimated with linearization, 0.116.

```
1    PROC RATIO DATA = EXCZ12_4 FILETYPE=SAS DESIGN=JACKKNIFE;
2    NEST _ONE_;
3    WEIGHT W;
4    SETENV DECWIDTH=3;
5    NUMER OVPAYMNT;

Opened SAS data file C:\PROGRAM
FILES\SUDAAN\RELEASE801\EXAMPLES\STANDALONE\EXCZ12_4.SSD for reading.

6    DENOM PAYMENT;

Number of observations read     :     10     Weighted count :        65
Denominator degrees of freedom :      9


Variance Estimation Method: Delete-1 Jackknife
by: Variable, One.

-----------------------------------------------------
|                  |          |       |
| Variable         |          |       | One
|                  |          |       | 1          |
-----------------------------------------------------
|                  |          |       |            |
| OVPAYMNT/PAYME-  | Sample Size      |     10.000 |
| NT               | Weighted Size    |     65.000 |
|                  | Weighted X-Sum   |  17914.000 |
|                  | Weighted Y-Sum   |   6922.500 |
|                  | Ratio Est.       |      0.386 |
|                  | SE Ratio         |      0.132 |
-----------------------------------------------------

RATIO used
```

Chapter Thirteen – Solutions

13.1 *In a community containing 200 households, it is desired to conduct a mail survey for purposes of estimating X (the number of persons 18-64 years of age in the community), R_1 (the proportion of employed persons among all persons 18-64 years of age), and R_2 (the average number of work days lost per employed person per year among employed persons 18-64 years old). From a collection of ten households in a nearby similar community, the accompanying data were obtained. How large a sample is needed in order to be virtually certain of estimating X to within 20%, R_1 to within 30%, and R_2 to within 25%?*

Household	Persons 18-64 Years	Employed Persons 18-64 Years	Work Days Lost in Past Month
a	4	3	1
b	2	1	1
c	3	2	2
d	1	0	0
e	1	1	2
f	0	0	0
g	2	2	3
h	5	4	2
i	0	0	0
j	2	1	2

Solution: This is a simple one-stage cluster sampling design, therefore the formulas for sample size that were presented in Chapter 9 will be used.

The sample size formula for estimating a total, X, is the following.

$$m = \frac{z_{1-\alpha/2}^2 * M * \hat{V}_{1x}^2}{z_{1-\alpha/2}^2 * \hat{V}_{1x}^2 + (M-1) * \varepsilon^2}$$

$$\hat{V}_{1x}^2 = \frac{\hat{\sigma}_{1x}^2}{\bar{x}^2}$$

Let $M = 200, z_{1-\alpha/2} = 3, and \ \varepsilon = 0.2$

STATA can be used to compute the mean and standard deviation from the sample data.

```
. sum adults

    Variable |      Obs       Mean   Std. Dev.        Min        Max
-------------+--------------------------------------------------------
      adults |       10          2   1.632993          0          5
```

$$m = \frac{z_{1-\alpha/2}^2 * M * \hat{V}_{1x}^2}{z_{1-\alpha/2}^2 * \hat{V}_{1x}^2 + (M-1) * \varepsilon^2}$$

$$\hat{V}_{1x}^2 = \frac{\hat{\sigma}_{1x}^2}{\bar{x}^2} = \frac{1.633^2}{2^2} = 0.667$$

$$m = \frac{3^2 * 200 * 0.667}{3^2 * 0.667 + 199 * 0.2^2} = 85.96$$

The required number of households for estimating the total number of adults to within 20% is 86.

The sample size for R_1 can be estimated using the formula for a ratio estimate. Again, from Chapter 9, the formula is the following.

$$m = \frac{z_{1-\alpha/2}^2 * M * \hat{V}_{1R}^2}{z_{1-\alpha/2}^2 * \hat{V}_{1R}^2 + (M-1) * \varepsilon^2}$$

$$\hat{V}_{1R}^2 = \frac{\hat{\sigma}_{1x}^2}{\bar{x}^2} + \frac{\hat{\sigma}_{1y}^2}{\bar{y}^2} - \left(2 * \frac{\hat{\sigma}_{1xy}}{\bar{x}\bar{y}}\right)$$

STATA can be used to compute the information required for this sample size calculation. First,
$$\hat{V}_{1R}^2$$
has to be estimated. To do this, we need the mean and variances for the variables adults and employed. The covariance between adults and employed can be calculated using the `correlate` function in STATA with the covariance option.

```
. sum adults employed

    Variable |      Obs        Mean   Std. Dev.        Min        Max
-------------+-----------------------------------------------------------
      adults |       10           2   1.632993          0          5
    employed |       10         1.4   1.349897          0          4


. correlate adults employed, covariance
(obs=10)

             |   adults  employed
-------------+------------------
      adults |  2.66667
    employed |  2.11111   1.82222
```

$$\hat{V}_{1R}^2 = \frac{\hat{\sigma}_{1x}^2}{\bar{x}^2} + \frac{\hat{\sigma}_{1y}^2}{\bar{y}^2} - \left(2 * \frac{\hat{\sigma}_{1xy}}{\overline{xy}}\right) = \frac{2.6667}{2^2} + \frac{1.8222}{1.4^2} - \left(2 * \frac{2.1111}{2 * 1.4}\right) = 0.0884$$

$$m = \frac{3^2 * 200 * 0.0884}{3^2 * 0.0884 + 199 * 0.3^2} = 8.507$$

The required number of households for estimating the total number of employed adults to within 30% is 9.

This sample size for R_2 can be estimated using the sample size formula for estimating a ratio. First, we need to compute a variable that is the average number of days lost per employed adult in each household.

```
. gen daylstyr = dayslost*12

. sum employed daylstyr

    Variable |      Obs        Mean   Std. Dev.        Min        Max
-------------+-----------------------------------------------------------
    employed |       10         1.4   1.349897          0          4
    daylstyr |       10        15.6    12.7122          0         36


. correlate  employed  daylstyr, covariance
(obs=10)

             | employed daylstyr
-------------+------------------
    employed |  1.82222
    daylstyr |     10.4      161.6
```

$$\hat{V}_{1R}^2 = \frac{\hat{\sigma}_{1x}^2}{\bar{x}^2} + \frac{\hat{\sigma}_{1y}^2}{\bar{y}^2} - \left(2 * \frac{\hat{\sigma}_{1xy}}{\overline{xy}}\right) = \frac{1.8222}{1.4^2} + \frac{161.6}{15.6^2} - \left(2 * \frac{10.4}{1.4 * 15.6}\right) = 0.6413$$

$$m = \frac{3^2 * 200 * 0.6413}{3^2 * 0.6413 + 199 * 0.25^2} = 63.39$$

The sample size required to estimate the average number of days lost per employed adult is 64. **Note**: this estimate differs from the sample size reported in the back of the book.

The sample size should be 86, which is the largest size calculated for the three desired estimates.

13.2   *For the data of Exercise 13.1 assume that 20% of the population would not respond to the questionnaire. Assume further that it costs $1.50 per questionnaire for the initial mailing, $10.00 per questionnaire for the processing of mailed questionnaires, and $60.00 per interview (cost of obtaining the interview and processing the data) for nonrespondents. Determine the proportion of nonrespondents that should be sampled and the total number of initial questionnaires that should be mailed.*

Solution: The proportion of nonrespondents that should be sampled is given by

$$\left(\frac{C_0 + C_1 P_1}{C_2 P_1}\right)^{1/2} = \left(\frac{1.5 + 10 * 0.8}{60 * 0.8}\right)^{1/2} = 0.44$$

From the nonrespondents, 44% should be sampled.

The number of initial questionnaires that should be sent is given by Equation 13.5.

$$n = n'\left\{1 + (1 - P_1)\left[\left(\frac{C_2 P_1}{C_0 + C_1 P_1}\right)^{1/2} - 1\right]\right\}$$

$$= 86 * \left\{1 + (0.2)\left[\left(\frac{180 * 0.8}{4.5 + 30 * 0.8}\right)^{1/2} - 1\right]\right\} = 107.46$$

The number of initial questionnaires that should be sent is 108.

13.3   *Pick a simple random sample of the required number of households (as calculated in Exercise 13.2), and from the data given in Tables 13.2 and 13.3, using the appropriate sampling of nonrespondents, estimate X, R_1, and R_2.*

Solution: From Exercise 13.2, we know that 44% of nonrespondents should be sampled. There are 50 households with missing data, therefore 22 of them should be sampled. The sample command in STATA can be used to randomly select the households. Then, examine the list and use these true values to fill in the missing data in Table 13.2.

```
. sample 44
(28 observations deleted)

. list

        househld       adults      employed      wlssdays
  1.         42            1            1             0
  2.        113            3            3             2
  3.         26            2            2             1
  4.        144            1            1             1
  5.        165            1            1             0
  6.         21            3            2             0
  7.        173            2            2             2
  8.         88            3            3             1
  9.          3            3            2             2
 10.        182            2            2             0
 11.         68            1            1             0
 12.        176            3            3             2
 13.        129            2            2             2
 14.         36            1            1             1
 15.        177            2            1             0
 16.         75            2            2             2
 17.         79            2            2             2
 18.        155            1            1             1
 19.        190            3            3             1
 20.        191            2            1             1
 21.         89            1            1             0
 22.        105            2            2             1
```

Next, we use the survey procedures in STATA to estimate X, R_1, and R_2.

```
. gen M = 200

. gen wt = M / 172

. svyset household [pweight=wt], fpc(M)

        pweight: wt
            VCE: linearized
    Single unit: missing
        Strata 1: <one>
           SU 1: household
          FPC 1: M


. svy: total adults
(running total on estimation sample)

Survey: Total estimation

Number of strata =          1      Number of obs   =      172
Number of PSUs   =        172      Population size =      200
                                   Design df       =      171


------------------------------------------------------------
               |               Linearized
               |      Total    Std. Err.    [95% Conf. Interval]
---------------+--------------------------------------------
        adults |   513.9535     8.57466      497.0277   530.8793
------------------------------------------------------------
```

The estimated total number of adults in this community is 513.9 or 514. The standard error of this estimate is 8.6.

```
. svy: ratio  employed adults
(running ratio on estimation sample)

Survey: Ratio estimation

Number of strata =          1      Number of obs   =      172
Number of PSUs   =        172      Population size =      200
                                   Design df       =      171


    _ratio_1: employed/adults


------------------------------------------------------------
               |               Linearized
               |      Ratio    Std. Err.    [95% Conf. Interval]
---------------+--------------------------------------------
      _ratio_1 |   .5135747    .0107925      .492271   .5348783
------------------------------------------------------------
```

The estimated proportion of employed adults between the ages of 18 and 64 is 0.51. The standard error of this estimate is 0.01.

```
. svy: ratio daylstyr employed
(running ratio on estimation sample)

Survey: Ratio estimation

Number of strata =          1        Number of obs    =       172
Number of PSUs    =      172        Population size  =       200
                                    Design df        =       171

       _ratio_1: daylstyr/employed


-----------------------------------------------------------------
              |                Linearized
              |       Ratio    Std. Err.    [95% Conf. Interval]
--------------+--------------------------------------------------
     _ratio_1 |    10.30837    .2338656     9.846735     10.77001
-----------------------------------------------------------------
```

The estimated number of days lost per employed person per year is 10.3. The standard error of this estimate is 0.23.

13.4   *Consider the data presented in the example used to illustrate the hot deck method. Impute the missing values for MMSE using the hot deck method as used in that example with the following modification. Assume that the individuals with missing values will in general have lower MMSEs than those who had measured values on this variable. To take this into consideration, use as an imputed value 80% of the value taken from the hot deck method. How does the resulting estimated mean and its standard error compare with that obtained from the hot deck method without this modification?*

Solution: Suppose there is additional information about the sampling design. Let us assume that this is a simple random sample and that we are sampling a small fraction of the total population. We can use the `summary` command in STATA to compute the estimated mean and standard deviation for the data using the hot deck method as in the example, and our modification of the hot deck method.

```
. sum MMSE

    Variable |     Obs       Mean    Std. Dev.      Min        Max
-------------+---------------------------------------------------
        MMSE |      20       18.8     4.990517       11         27

. display 4.990517 / sqrt(20)
1.1159135

. sum MMSE_80

    Variable |     Obs       Mean    Std. Dev.      Min        Max
```

```
-------------+----------------------------------------------------------------
      MMSE_80 |        20        18.1     5.077297              9           27

. display 5.077297 / sqrt(20)
1.1353181
```

The estimated mean and standard error from the hot deck method in the illustrative example are 18.8 and 1.12. The corresponding estimates from our modification of the hot deck method are 18.1 and 1.14. The estimated mean is slightly smaller, but the standard error change was minimal.

13.5   *Repeat the illustrative example presented in Section 13.6 with the modification discussed in Exercise 13.4. How does the estimated mean and its standard error computed on the basis of multiple imputation compare with that originally obtained?*

Solution: STATA can be used to calculate the means and standard deviations for the three MMSE combinations. Then, the equations presented in Section 13.6 can be used to combine these three estimates to obtain a mean and standard error from multiple imputation.

```
. sum MMSE_1 MMSE_2 MMSE_3

    Variable |      Obs        Mean    Std. Dev.        Min         Max
-------------+----------------------------------------------------------------
      MMSE_1 |       20       18.25    5.035401           9          27
      MMSE_2 |       20        18.5    4.968321          10          27
      MMSE_3 |       20        18.6    4.805698          11          27

. display 5.035401 / sqrt(20)
1.1259499

. display 4.968321 / sqrt(20)
1.1109503

. display 4.805698 / sqrt(20)
1.0745867
```

$$s_w^2 = \frac{1.125^2 + 1.111^2 + 1.075^2}{3} = 1.219$$

$$s_b^2 = \frac{\left(1 + \frac{1}{k}\right)\sum_{i=1}^k (\bar{x}_i - \bar{x})^2}{(k-1)} = \frac{\frac{4}{3}[0.04 + 0.0025 + 0.0225]}{2} = 0.0433$$

$$\bar{x} = \frac{18.25 + 18.5 + 18.6}{3} = 18.45$$

$$\widehat{Var}(\bar{x}) = 0.0433 + 1.219 = 1.2623$$

$$\widehat{SE}(\bar{x}) = 1.124$$

The estimated mean from this modification of the example in Section 13.6 is smaller, which is expected because the imputed values in this exercise were 80% of those used in the book. The standard error is slightly smaller from this modification, and is more similar to the three individual estimates. The reason the standard error is smaller with this modification is because two of the values that were imputed were initially extreme, 26 and 27. With the modification, these imputed values were replaced with 21 and 22, respectively, and these values are closer to the center of the distribution of the observed data. Therefore, the resulting three means were more similar with this modification, and hence the between imputation contribution to the standard error was lower.

13.6 *Use the hot deck method to impute missing values for the data in Table 13.2. How does the resulting estimated mean and its standard error compare with that which would have been obtained had there been 100% response?*

Solution: For this problem, we have the data for the entire population and we will compare the true population mean number of lost work days to the estimates obtained from the incomplete data (based on 150 households) and the hot deck imputed data set. We can use the summary procedure in STATA to compute the means, standard deviations, and standard errors.

Incomplete Sample – Based on 150 households

```
. sum wlssdays

    Variable |      Obs        Mean    Std. Dev.       Min        Max
-------------+-----------------------------------------------------------
    wlssdays |      150    1.166667    1.476513          0          6

. display 1.47651 / sqrt(150)
.12055654
```

Imputed data using hot deck method – 200 households

```
. sum wlssdays

    Variable |      Obs        Mean    Std. Dev.       Min        Max
-------------+-----------------------------------------------------------
    wlssdays |      200       1.145    1.484924          0          6

. display 1.48492 / sqrt(200)
.1049997
```

True values – Entire population

```
. sum wlssdays

    Variable |      Obs        Mean    Std. Dev.       Min        Max
-------------+-----------------------------------------------------------
    wlssdays |      200       1.115    1.345671          0          6

. display 1.34567 / sqrt(200)
.09515324
```

The estimate of the mean number of lost work days is biased upward for both the incomplete data and the hot deck imputed data, although the imputed data has an estimate that is closer to the truth. Hence, the imputed data mean is less biased compared to the incomplete data. The standard error computed using the imputed data is smaller (and closer to the true data standard error) than the standard error computed using the incomplete data. This is expected since the incomplete data set had 50 fewer observations.

Chapter Fourteen – Solutions

14.1   *A simple random sample was taken of 525 workers in a plant employing 3575 workers. All persons sampled were given an electrocardiogram which was read for abnormalities independently by two physicians. Of the 525 sample persons, 25 had abnormalities noted by both physicians; 15 had abnormalities noted by physician A, but not by physician B; 37 had abnormalities noted by physician B only; and the remainder had no abnormalities noted by either physician. Based on these data, what would be the estimated number of abnormalities among the 3575 workers?*

Solution: This exercise is an example of a dual samples problem. Equation 14.9 can be used to estimate the number of abnormalities among the 3575 workers.

		Physician A		
		Yes	No	
Physician B	Yes	25	37	62
	No	15		
		40		

$$\hat{n} = \frac{40 * 62}{25} = 99.2$$

$$\hat{N} = 99.2 * \frac{N}{n} = 675.6 = 676$$

14.2   *The same persons were screened for diabetes on the basis of a single fasting blood glucose test. The particular screening method has a known sensitivity equal to 80% and a specificity equal to 96%. Based on findings of 14 positive tests, estimate and give 95% confidence intervals for the prevalence of diabetes among these employees.*

Solution: Equations 14.5 and 14.6 can be used to estimate the prevalence and the standard error of the prevalence of diabetes among these employees.

$$\hat{\pi} = \frac{\hat{p} + S_p - 1}{S_e + S_p - 1} = \frac{0.027 + 0.96 - 1}{0.80 + 0.96 - 1} = -0.017$$

This negative estimate indicates that the screening test is bad. When we examine the numerator we see that the estimated prevalence, p, of a positive test is less than $(1-S_p)$, which is the probability that a person who truly does not have the disease will have a positive test. In other words, the probability of a random person from the population testing positive is less than the probability of a known non-diseased person being positive. Because this estimate is negative, it does not make sense to construct a 95% confidence interval.

14.3   *These same persons were also screened for hypertension by use of a standard sphygmomanometer examination and, based on this examination, 63 were positive. Of those screened as positive, 25 were given more intensive evaluation for hypertension, and 21 were confirmed as being hypertensive. A sample of 50 persons was taken from those originally screened as negative, and 8 of these were found on the more intensive evaluation to be hypertensive. Based on these findings, what is the estimated prevalence of hypertension in this population? Give 95% confidence intervals for this estimated proportion.*

Solution: Equations 14.7 and 14.8 can be used to estimate the prevalence and standard error of the prevalence of hypertension among these employees.

$$\hat{\pi} = \frac{\frac{k_1}{m_1} * m + \frac{k_2}{m_2} * (n-m)}{n} = \frac{\frac{21}{25} * 63 + \frac{8}{50} * (462)}{525} = 0.2416$$

$$\widehat{Var}(\hat{\pi}) = \left(\frac{k_1}{m_1} - \frac{k_2}{m_2}\right)^2 * \frac{\frac{m}{n}\left(1-\frac{m}{n}\right)}{n} + \left(\frac{m}{n}\right)^2 \frac{\frac{k_1}{m_1}\left(1-\frac{k_1}{m_1}\right)}{m_1} + \left(1-\frac{m}{n}\right)^2 \frac{\frac{k_2}{m_2}\left(1-\frac{k_2}{m_2}\right)}{m_2}$$

$$= \left(\frac{21}{25} - \frac{8}{50}\right)^2 * \frac{\frac{63}{525}\left(1-\frac{63}{525}\right)}{525} + \left(\frac{63}{525}\right)^2 * \frac{\frac{21}{25}\left(1-\frac{21}{25}\right)}{25}$$

$$+ \left(1-\frac{63}{525}\right)^2 \frac{\frac{8}{50}\left(1-\frac{8}{50}\right)}{50}$$

$$= (0.4624 * 0.000201) + 0.0000774 + 0.0020816 = 0.00225$$

$$\widehat{SE}(\hat{\pi}) = 0.0475$$

$$95\% \ CI = 0.2416 \pm 1.96(0.0475) = 0.2416 \pm 0.0930 = (0.1486, 0.3346)$$

14.4 *From the data presented in the previous exercise, estimate the sensitivity and the specificity of the sphygmomanometer examination used in the screening for hypertension.*

Solution: Equations 14.9 and 14.10 can be used to estimate the sensitivity and specificity of the sphygmomanometer examination.

$$\hat{S}_e = \frac{m \frac{k_1}{m_1}}{m\left(\frac{k_1}{m_1} - \frac{k_2}{m_2}\right) + n\frac{k_2}{m_2}} = \frac{63\frac{21}{25}}{63\left(\frac{21}{25} - \frac{8}{50}\right) + n\frac{8}{50}} = \frac{52.92}{42.84 + 84} = 0.42$$

$$\hat{S}_p = \frac{(n-m)(1 - \frac{k_2}{m_2})}{m\left(\frac{k_2}{m_2} - \frac{k_1}{m_1}\right) + n(1 - \frac{k_2}{m_2})} = \frac{(462)(1 - \frac{8}{50})}{63\left(\frac{8}{50} - \frac{21}{25}\right) + 525(1 - \frac{8}{50})} = \frac{388.08}{-42.84 + 441}$$
$$= 0.97$$

The estimated sensitivity is 0.42 and the estimated specificity is 0.97.

14.5 *A simple random sample was taken of 300 households in a community containing 3562 households. Respondents from each household were queried on whether there had been a burglary during the past year in either that house or any other house on the block segment containing that house. The following six (6) burglaries were reported:*

Burglary	Number of Households Eligible to Report the Burglary
1	3
2	2
3	7
4	6
5	8
6	2

Based on these findings, estimate the number of burglaries that occurred in that community over the past year.

Solution: We will use the procedures outlined in Section 14.5 in the book to solve this problem.

$$x'_{mult} = \left(\frac{N}{n}\right) x^*$$

$$x^* = \frac{1}{6} + \frac{1}{2} + \frac{1}{7} + \frac{1}{6} + \frac{1}{8} + \frac{1}{2} = 1.6011$$

$$x'_{mult} = \left(\frac{N}{n}\right) x^* = \left(\frac{3562}{300}\right) 1.6011 = 19.01$$

Using all of the information contained in the sample, the estimated number of robberies is about 19. **Note:** if we had used the conventional counting rule, then:

$$x' = \left(\frac{3562}{300}\right) 600 = 71.24$$

This estimate is much larger than the one we obtained using network sampling.

Chapter Fifteen – Solutions

15.1   *A newspaper wants to conduct a national omnibus survey on a variety of issues, including politics, the environment, taxes, and foreign affairs. They want 2,000 completed interviews in the shortest time possible and therefore want to use the most efficient, quick turn-around sampling strategy that will still allow the results to be statistically valid. What approach should the newspaper use? What is the final response rate using the minimum response rate (American Association for Public Opinion Research Response Rate calculation #1) if the final distribution of cases is as follows:*

> *Completed Interviews (I) =2,000*
> *Partially completed interviews (P) = 36*
> *Refusals & breakoffs (R) = 962*
> *Noncontatcts (NC) = 1,203*
> *Other cases (O) = 38*
> *Unknown if household (UH) = 1,249*
> *Unknown other (UO) = 12*

Solution: The minimum response rate will be as follows:

$$Minimum\ response\ rate = \frac{I}{(I+P)+(R+NC+O)+(UH+UO)}$$
$$= \frac{2,000}{(2,000+36)+(962+1,203+38)+(1,249+12)} = \frac{2,000}{5,500}$$
$$= 0.3636$$

15.2   *The state of Georgia wants to conduct a random digit dialed telephone survey of the general adult population on topics related to education. They want to complete 3,000 interviews with Hispanic households. What starting sample size is required if the following sample assumptions are used:*

> *Non-working household number rate = 32.6%*
> *Eligibility rate = 17.1%*
> *Non-response after eligibility = 54.3%*

Solution: The survey starting sample size will be 56,957 telephone numbers. Use the following basic formula for calculating the starting sample size (n) given the stated assumptions.

$$n*(working\ household\ rate)*(eligibility\ rate)$$
$$*(cooperation\ after\ eligibility\ rate) = completes$$

Therefore:

$$n = \frac{3,000}{(1.0 - 0.326) * (0.171) * (1.0 - 0.543)} = 56,957$$

15.3   A health planning group wants to conduct a telephone survey on issues related to health insurance coverage and access to medical care in New Mexico. They want to complete 2.400 random digit dialed interviews with an equal distribution of completed interviews in four policy planning areas (the four areas are based on contiguous counties but are not equivalent in terms of population distribution). Given the following sampling assumptions, what are te starting sample sizes required for each of the 4 policy planning areas and what is the total amount of sample required overall?

Assumption	Area #1	Area #2	Area #3	Area #4
% working household numbers	76.4	66.2	72.9	69.3
% eligibility	96.2	95.3	97.2	96.3
% cooperation after eligibility	44.6	39.8	42.7	46.5

Solution: The project will require a total sample of 8.136 numbers (Area 1=1,830; Area 2=2,390; Area 3=1,983; and Area 4=1,933). Calculate the required sample for each area, then sum across the areas to determine the total sample required. Use the following formula:

$$n * (working\ household\ rate) * (eligibility\ rate)$$
$$* (cooperation\ after\ eligibility\ rate) = completes$$

Area 1:

$$n_{Area\ 1} = \frac{600}{(0.764) * (0.962) * (0.446)} = 1,830$$

Area 2:

$$n_{Area\ 2} = \frac{600}{(0.662) * (0.953) * (0.398)} = 2,390$$

Area 3:

$$n_{Area\ 3} = \frac{600}{(0.729) * (0.972) * (0.427)} = 1,983$$

Area 4:

$$n_{Area\ 4} = \frac{600}{(0.693) * (0.963) * (0.465)} = 1,933$$

Printed in the USA
CPSIA information can be obtained
at www.ICGtesting.com
CBHW080128141024
15713CB00007B/14